MW01235539

HYPNOTIC GASTRIC BAND

© Copyright 2020 by

All rights reserved.

This document is geared towards providing exact and reliable information with regards to the topic and issue covered. The publication is sold with the idea that the publisher is not required to render accounting, officially permitted, or otherwise, qualified services. If advice is necessary, legal or professional, a practiced individual in the profession should be ordered.

From a Declaration of Principles which was accepted and approved equally by a Committee of the American Bar Association and a Committee of Publishers and Associations.

In no way is it legal to reproduce, duplicate, or transmit any part of this document in either electronic means or in printed format. Recording of this publication is strictly prohibited and any storage of this document is not allowed unless with written permission from the publisher. All rights reserved.

The information provided herein is stated to be truthful and consistent, in that any liability, in terms of inattention or otherwise, by any usage or abuse of any policies, processes, or directions contained within is the solitary and utter responsibility of the recipient reader. Under no circumstances will any legal responsibility or blame be held against the publisher for any reparation, damages, or monetary loss due to the information herein, either directly or indirectly.

Respective authors own all copyrights not held by the publisher.

The information herein is offered for informational purposes solely, and is universal as so. The presentation of the information is without contract or any type of guarantee assurance.

The trademarks that are used are without any consent, and the publication of the trademark is without permission or backing by the trademark owner. All trademarks and brands within this book are for clarifying purposes only and are the owned by the owners themselves, not affiliated with this document.

TABLE OF CONTENT

INTRODUCTION

For decades, the idea of losing weight by hypnosis has been around, but now some hypnotherapists propose "gastric bypass hypnosis," often called "lap band hypnosis." This "procedure" is performed to "reprogram" patients' minds to assume that their stomachs are smaller, leaving them unable to eat big meals without feeling uncomfortably full.

More than 200,000 Americans undergo invasive and costly surgical procedures each year to remove, reposition or constrict parts of their stomachs. These treatments can cost up to $35,000, but gastric bypass hypnotherapists say that their hypnosis sessions can provide far less money for equivalent weight loss results: around $1,200.

Certified hypnotherapist Rena Greenberg said that in the past 20 years, she has consulted with over 100,000 patients and is confident that hypnosis helps keep her customers from obsessing over food.

Chapter 1: UNDERSTANDING HYPNOSIS

What about hypnosis?
Hypnosis is a trance-like mental condition in which people are subjected to increased concentration, focus, and suggestibility. Although hypnosis is often described as a sleeping state, it is better represented as a state of intense attention, increased suggestibility, and vivid fantasies. In a hypnotic state, people sometimes seem sleepy and zoned out, but they are in a state of hyper-awareness.
Hypnosis is a very real method used as a therapeutic technique, but many myths and misconceptions exist. Hypnosis has been shown to have medical and psychological effects, mainly to reduce pain and anxiety. It has also been proposed that hypnosis may decrease the symptoms of dementia.

FORMS OF HYPNOSIS
There are a few distinct forms of hypnosis administration:
Directed hypnosis: This type of hypnosis includes using tools, such as recorded instructions and music, to induce a hypnotic state. Web sites and mobile apps mostly use this method of hypnosis.
Hypnotherapy: In psychotherapy, hypnotherapy is hypnosis and is used by licensed clinicians and psychologists to treat depression, anxiety, post-traumatic stress disorder (PTSD), and eating disorders.
Self-hypnosis: Self-hypnosis is a process that happens when an individual is self-induced by a hypnotic state. For pain relief or stress management, it is also used as a self-help tool.
Utilizations

Why should a person decide to try hypnosis? In certain cases, to help cope with chronic pain or relieve pain and anxiety caused by medical procedures such as surgery or childbirth, people may seek hypnosis.

The following are only a few of the hypnosis applications that have been seen through research:

- Alleviation of irritable bowel syndrome (IBS) related symptoms
- Pain management during dental procedures
- Elimination or elimination, including warts and psoriasis, of skin conditions
- Control of such ADHD symptoms
- Treatment of problems with chronic pain such as rheumatoid arthritis
- Treatment and pain relief during childbirth 4
- Reduction in signs of dementia
- Reduction of nausea and vomiting of patients with cancer who undergo chemotherapy

Hypnosis has also been used to assist individuals with behavior improvements, such as stopping smoking, losing weight, or avoiding bed-wetting.

Potential Pitfalls

Having misunderstandings about the subject of hypnosis is common.

While amnesia can occur in extremely rare cases, people typically remember everything that occurred when hypnotized. However, hypnosis can have a significant effect on memory. Posthypnotic amnesia may lead an individual to forget certain items that occurred before or during hypnosis. This effect is, however, usually limited and temporary.

The effects of mass media have been greatly underestimated, while hypnosis can be used to enhance memory. Research has shown that hypnosis does not contribute to a meaningful improvement or memory continuity, and hypnosis can lead to false or distorted memories.

Despite stories about hypnotized people without their consent, hypnosis involves voluntary intervention on the part of the patient. In terms of how hypnotizable and suggestible they are while under hypnosis, people vary. Research suggests that highly suggestive people are more likely to experience a diminished sense of agency when under hypnosis.

While people frequently assume that their actions under hypnosis appear to occur beyond the force of their will, a hypnotist can not make you perform things against your wishes.

While hypnosis may improve outcomes, it does not make individuals stronger or more athletic than their current physical abilities.

The History Of Hypnosis

The use of hypnotic-like trance states dates back thousands of years, but during the late 18th century, hypnosis began to originate from a doctor named Franz Mesmer. The operation got off to a poor start due to Mesmer's spiritual values, but the focus eventually shifted to a more scientific approach.

Hypnotism became more important in psychology in the late 19th century and was used by Jean-Martin Charcot to treat women suffering from what was then known as hysteria. This work influenced Sigmund Freud and the development of psychoanalysis.

More recently, there have been several different theories to describe exactly how hypnosis works. One of the best-known theories is Hilgard's neo-dissociation theory of hypnosis.

According to Hilgard, individuals in a hypnotic state experience a split consciousness in which there are two different origins of mental activity. While one stream of consciousness reacts to the hypnotist's suggestions, another dissociated stream processes information outside the hypnotized person's conscious awareness.

Losing weight can be a difficult challenge that is not made any easier and often dangerous by the conflicting advice out there in the world. We are continually bombarded with TV shows, advertisements, and social media feeds full of food images. The presence of these can make the temptation to turn away from healthy or intuitive eating very strong.

Then there are weight loss pills and other commercial weight management programs that focus on minimizing what you eat rather than looking at how you eat or what you think about the food you put in your body. It is no wonder that around what we put in our bodies, many damaging mindsets have developed.

Hypnosis of weight loss can be a good way of challenging these mental habits and temptation times, helping you to live a healthier life.

The goal of hypnotherapy for weight loss is to make you feel good about your body, change unhealthy thoughts about food, and help you lose weight responsibly without impacting your emotional well-being. By engaging the unconscious mind with powerful suggestion strategies, a hypnotherapist will help you develop a healthy relationship with food and exercise, which is important for safe weight loss and long-term weight management.

Is losing weight important to me?

Many individuals insist that they ought to lose weight, whether they are overweight or not. But the fact is, very few people are happy with the shape and size of their bodies, irrespective of whether they need to lose weight.

You will find more information on weight loss at Nutritionist Resource.

Trust in the body

While people must lose weight if, for health reasons, they are overweight, it is not good to feel ashamed of the need or desire to lose weight. Since body shape and size are so linked to the Western concept of beauty, people are constantly trying to cut corners for 'quick fixes.'

Weight loss supplements, fad diets, and grueling exercise routines are ways people want to lose weight. What do you have to ask yourself: am I pleased to do this? Will I continue doing this for the remainder of my life?

This is where hypnotherapy for weight loss can improve. To change your body, you need first to change your mind. Why am I unhappy with my body, and why am I not able to lose weight? You have to ask yourself.

To read more about how low self-confidence can be boosted by hypnotherapy, visit our fact sheet.

How does hypnosis for weight loss work?

Weight loss hypnotherapy is becoming more common, and for people all over the world, it is ideal for maintaining a healthy weight in the long term.

Over time, you'll learn how to replace your negative patterns with healthier behaviors suggested by your hypnotherapist- and a series of hypnotherapy sessions for weight loss.

What happens during hypnosis for weight loss?

Your hypnotherapist will lead you into a state of deep relaxation.

When your body and mind are fully relaxed, your hypnotherapist will enter your unconscious mind (the part of us that operates all the time but we are not aware of, i.e., instincts and survival mechanisms).

To explain why a client overeats and suggests new ways of thinking through visualizations, soothing, carefully worded scripts may be used. You should ignore any suggestions that you do not feel comfortable with without any feedback from your hypnotherapist. See below for some of the techniques and visualizations that they may use.

HYPNOTHERAPY FOR WEIGHT REDUCTION STRATEGIES

While each situation is different and everybody has their reasons for wanting to lose weight, there are some suggestions you might find:

- Imagine the body you want or the level of fitness/wellness you want to achieve.
- Imagining how you'd feel about your new look and well-being.
- Imagining yourself hitting the goal comfortably.
- See how far you have shifted from now.
- Imagine how energized you would feel and how safe.

Realizing that the more you exercise, the more you want to exercise, and the more difficult it will become to do so. Such techniques are intended to encourage you so that you can take control of your decisions. However, if you're concerned that your relationship with certain types of food is becoming unhealthy, hypnotherapy for food addiction could help you break these negative thought cycles.

Via weight loss hypnosis, you can learn to enjoy the taste of nutritious food and resist wanting sugary, unhealthy foods. To respect your body, you can also learn not to see it as a source of distress. By addressing those deep feelings that shape the foundations of your eating habits, hypnosis for weight loss will help you adopt a healthier lifestyle and a happier attitude.

Your Weight Loss Possible Blocks

For several factors, many people try and fail to lose weight. Sometimes referred to as 'secondary advantages,' these triggers are largely implicit, making it difficult for us to overcome them.

When anyone loses weight, it is worth looking at the confidence that kept the weight in place for so long. We still hold convictions on two levels; we think at the conscious level of optimistic thoughts about ourselves, our worth, and what we deserve as human beings, but our actions unconsciously give away our emotional beliefs.

A clinical hypnotherapist, Amreeta Chapman/Aujayeb, addresses the challenges people can face while losing weight. The truth is, we can often gain protection by not making changes-we feel secure staying just as we are. So, we may actively want to lose weight, but something in the subconscious stops us from making it a reality. Hypnotherapy for weight loss aims to discover these factors, allowing consumers to finally break through barriers that may have kept them from losing weight for many years.

You eat consolation from food

When we are children, we learn to associate feeding with the comfort of our mothers. Some experts claim that this bond never really leaves us, so when life gets stressful, we can return to those early days of utter dependency. This is where emotional eating can become a concern.

If you've ever found yourself reaching for a chocolate bar after a long day or ordering a takeaway when you're feeling lonely and sad, then you could be a comfort eater. As a comfort eater, you will find it more difficult to lose weight because you have let food become your coping device, and without it, you do not know how to cope with your feelings.

Hypnotherapy will help remedy this, helping you understand how unpleasant emotions are treated in a manner that does not lead to eating comfort.

The biggest change is that I have been much less bothered to eat. I love it, but when my body is hungry, I have learned to eat, not only because my mind wants anything to soothe my feelings.

You're eating mindlessly,

To lose weight, you have to be honest about how much you eat and exercise. Even if you keep a food diary or use a food-tracking app, it's easy to forget about the occasional snack here and there. Maybe when you're making dinner, you select ingredients? Do you catch something at work on your trip, or do you tuck your afternoon tea into a biscuit?

These foods 'on the go' are always the ones that catch us out. They add up, however. Even if you stick to salad for dinner religiously, it's not going to do you any favors to easily neglect all the stuff you consume in between. This kind of mindless eating is something that hypnotherapy for weight loss will help you overcome.

Gastric band hypnotherapy might help you if you struggle with conscious eating. For longer, the goal is to make you feel fuller, which may help avoid unnecessary day-long grazing.

You're banning food

You're advised not to open them like a mystery package; it can make them all the more enticing by excluding certain foods from your diet. If you find yourself reducing the foods you eat, you're more likely to want to binge when your willpower dives.

The key to sustainable and successful weight loss is learning to eat attentively. If you eat carefully, savoring every bite, you will be able to enjoy your favorite foods in moderation and avoid putting on weight.

A critical feature of hypnosis of weight loss is motivating customers to consciously eat emotional factors and maintain a stable relationship with food that maintains a long-term, balanced weight.

You're not exercising enough,

Exercise is just as important as diet when it comes to weight loss. Mental blocks can also discourage us from wanting to work out, including:

- Feeling an absence of means
- Feeling too self-conscious to exercise publicly

- Convincing yourself that you can 'go tomorrow' (every day)

Weight loss hypnotherapy will help you break down the mental barriers that hinder your body from making the best of you. In general, it will make you feel better about yourself more often than not by keeping your body running and your heart beating, leading to healthier behaviors and long-term satisfaction.

Can hypnosis for weight loss work out for me?

One of the most commonly asked questions during hypnotherapy sessions is: does weight loss hypnotherapy work for me? The answer to that is, it is hard to say until you try it yourself. Although it certainly won't work the same way for everyone, the process of talking about building good habits and getting rid of bad habits will help to create a new level of awareness when it comes to diet and exercise. Hypnotherapy is a supportive procedure, an important thing to note, and a healthy diet plan and workout schedule can also be used. You will find it helpful to speak to your doctor or nutrition professional if you want advice about eating healthy and exercising. With all these dimensions, it is often a collective effort that leads to success.

Chapter 2: THE GASTRIC BAND HYPNOTHERAPY

A method used to help you lose weight is gastric band hypnotherapy. A hypnotherapist uses this technique to indicate to your subconscious that you have had a gastric band fitted around your stomach. Considered to be a non-invasive alternative to surgery for weight loss, a hypnotic gastric band may have many positive effects without the potential side effects.

One form of weight loss surgery often considered a last resort is a traditional gastric band. The band physically limits how much food you can eat by fitting a band around the upper part of your stomach, encouraging weight loss in many cases. Research has, however, shown that in the months and years following surgery, patients undergoing a physical gastric band face several complications, including the risk of slipping or eroding the band.

For those who have struggled with sustainable weight loss, diet changes, and weight-related problems, the often significant and sustained loss of weight that accompanies many gastric band procedures can be very attractive. It requires no surgery to have a 'virtual gastric band' fitted, also known as gastric band hypnotherapy.

A hypnotherapist can help you, on an unconscious level, to believe that you have had a physical procedure by working with your subconscious and that your stomach has decreased in size. No surgery or medication is used, making it an alternative that is safer and painless. We're going to discuss how this approach works, what it means, and how it can work for you.

What is a gastric band?

An adjustable silicone device used in surgery for weight loss is a gastric band. To create a small pouch above the device, the band is positioned around the upper section of your stomach. This limits the amount of food in your stomach that can be stored, making it difficult to eat large quantities.

A gastric band is one of the three weight-loss surgeries most commonly offered, available through private surgery, or for those with a BMI of 40 or more who meet specific criteria for an NHS procedure. A gastric band's main advantage is long-term, sustainable weight loss. It's still important to change your diet, exercise regularly, and attend post-surgery follow-up appointments to gain advice and support as needed for you to see the benefits.

A gastric band's goal is to limit food a person can eat physically, causing them to feel full of encouraging weight loss after eating very little. It is the last resort for most people who have this surgery after trying other weight loss methods. Fitting a gastric band, like any surgery, comes with risks.

- Some of the risks include if you have a physical gastric band:
- Slipping the band out of place. This can lead to nausea, vomiting, and heartburn. To readjust or remove the band, further surgery may be required.
- In your stomach, a leak. There is a small chance that food may leak into your tummy following a gastric bypass or gastric sleeve (another form of the gastric band), causing a serious infection that may require antibiotics and surgery to repair any damage.
- A gut that's blocked. Blockages may cause vomiting, tummy pain, difficulty swallowing, and bowel movement disorders. Blockages would have to be cleared by a specialist.
- Having malnutrition. After weight loss surgery, absorbing the right amount of vitamins and minerals

can become a problem, meaning that many will have to take lifetime supplements to avoid malnutrition risks.

- For 12-18 months post-surgery, women who have had a physical gastric band, sleeve, or bypass are also recommended to avoid becoming pregnant.
- But how do gastric physical bands vary from gastric band hypnosis? And can a gastrointestinal virtual band have the same benefits?

Hypnosis of the Gastric Band

Gastric band hypnosis can be used, without the complications that come with surgery, to help people lose weight. Many hypnotherapists employ a two-pronged approach. They first look at the root cause of your emotional eating to identify it.

HOW GASTRIC BAND HYPNOSIS FUNCTIONS

A hypnotherapist will put you in a state of hypnosis using relaxation techniques. Your subconscious is more open to suggestions in this relaxed state. Hypnotherapists make recommendations to your subconscious at this point. This suggestion is that you have a physical band fitted with gastric band hypnotherapy.

The mind is powerful, so your behavior will change accordingly if your subconscious accepts these suggestions. Typically, along with the 'fitting' of the virtual gastric band, confidence and behavior suggestions will be made to help you commit to this lifestyle change.

Many therapists will also teach self-hypnosis techniques to improve the work you have done following the session. It is also often advised to educate yourself on nutrition and exercise to promote physical health and well-being.

Chapter 3: GASTRIC BAND SURGERY

Gastric band surgery is a common form of weight loss (bariatric) surgery for severely overweight people (obese). It entails wrapping an elastic band around the top of your stomach, limiting how much you can consume. This helps you to lose weight.

How does a gastric band work?
When you have a gastric band, it creates a tiny pouch above the band at the top of your stomach. When you feed, this portion of your stomach fills up easily, allowing you to feel full faster and for longer than normal. This decreases the amount of food you consume, helps you lose weight.
Your surgeon can loosen or tighten the gastric band by injecting liquid into a tube attached to the band.
This influences the rate at which food moves from the pouch into the lower part of your stomach. This will ensure that you lose the necessary amount of weight over time.
The operation's success depends on you adopting a healthier lifestyle after the procedure, which involves improving your dietary habits and increasing your physical activity. This involves avoiding high-calorie beverages, such as alcohol, that are not limited by your gastric band.

Who can have a gastric band?
You must typically meet certain criteria to be eligible for gastric band surgery. These include:
- having a BMI (body mass index) of 40 or higher, or between 35 and 40 with a health condition like high blood pressure or diabetes

- having tried all other treatment options first, such as exercise and dieting
- being physically fit enough to undergo surgery and a general anesthetic
- committing to long-term follow-up, which includes routine check-ups and lifestyle changes
- being able to attend follow-up appointments daily

You may not be eligible for a gastric band if you have long-term health issues, such as inflammatory bowel disease, psychological disorder, or heart disease. You may need a psychological evaluation if you have any questions about your mental health.

If you're overweight, your GP can refer you to a specialized obesity treatment service to see if surgery may help. If you meet the above requirements, you may be eligible for gastric band surgery on the NHS; however, this depends on your local area's availability. Another option is to have the surgery done in a private location. Private surgery may be available in private hospitals or at some NHS centers.

Deciding on gastric band surgery

A gastric band is a serious treatment. It's important to know exactly what the operation entails and any possible complications and what to expect afterward.

If you're thinking of getting a gastric band, talk to your doctor about it. They'll also explore other weight-loss surgeries you might be able to do have, such as sleeve gastrectomy or a gastric bypass. Your surgeon will assist you in deciding what is best for you.

Here are some points to consider.

- A gastric band helps many people to lose weight. It can also help you prevent various health issues, such as high blood pressure, diabetes, and high cholesterol, or improve them if you already have them.

- The amount of weight lost varies from individual to individual, but most people lose about half of their excess weight in two years. Not everyone loses as much as they would like.
- Other forms of weight loss surgery might be safer in the long run, according to some evidence.
- It's likely that your gastric band will need to be replaced or removed, for example, if it slips or leaks.

Take the time to make sure you're happy with your decision to get a gastric band and ask your surgeon any questions you may have. If you want to proceed, you will be asked to sign a consent form, so make sure you are fully informed before signing.

Preparing for gastric band surgery
You will need to undergo some evaluations and blood tests to make sure you are fit for surgery. These can also
show whether you suffer from any health issues as a result of your obesity.
If you smoke, you'll be advised to quit - preferably at least 6 weeks before your surgery. Smoking has been shown to delay wound healing and increase the risk of complications. You may be asked to adopt a low-fat, low-carbohydrate diet for a period before your operation. This will help shrink the liver and make it safer and easier put the band in place.
A gastric band is done under general anesthesia, which implies you will be unconscious during the operation. You need to fast before having a general anesthetic. You will be given detailed instructions about when to quit drinking or eating. It's essential that you follow this advice.

On the day of your operation, the surgeon will speak to you to ensure that you are in good health and still willing to proceed. The medical staff will conduct any final examinations and prepare you for surgery. This could include prescribing compression stockings and/or administering an anticoagulant injection to avoid deep vein thrombosis (DVT).

What happens during gastric band surgery?
Your gastric band will be fitted using keyhole (laparoscopic) surgery. This means that instead of one big cut, the surgeon will conduct the operation with instruments implanted into multiple tiny cuts in your tummy (abdomen).
The band will be inserted and wrapped around the top of your stomach, forming a tiny pouch above the band. A fine tubing piece connects the band to an injection port, used to loosen or tighten the band. Your surgeon will stitch this into place, just under your skin. Your surgeon will then close the cut in your abdomen. This is usually done with dissolvable stitches, but it may also be done with clips removed in a week or so.

What To Expect Afterwards
At the hospital
You'll need to rest until the anesthetic wears off. You can also require pain medication to relieve any discomfort you may be feeling.
You will have a drip into a vein in your arm or hand to give you fluids until you are well enough to drink. You will be encouraged to get out of bed and walk about as soon as you can. This would reduce the chances of having a chest infection and the development of blood clots in your legs. Before you go home, your nurse will give you instructions about caring for your healing wounds and arranging a follow-up appointment.
Going home

You will be able to go home either that day or the next day after your surgery. Ensure that someone can transport you home and, if possible, stay with you for a day or two while the anesthetic wears off. You can continue to use over-the-counter pain relievers at home as required.

Because your gastric band will be partially filled (primed) during surgery, you will be limited on what you can eat right afterward. You won't be able to drink anything until after your operation. Your surgeon or dietitian will let you know when you will be able to start eating.

It can take a week or two for you to completely recover from gastric band surgery and resume your routine activities. However, since this differs from person to person, listening to the surgeon's advice is important.

After your surgery, you'll need to go for regular follow-up appointments to get your gastric band adjusted. This will ensure that you lose the necessary amount of weight over time.

Complications of gastric band surgery

Complications are problems that arise unexpectedly during or after the operation.

Any operation's potential complications include an unexpected reaction to the anesthetic, excessive bleeding, or a blood clot (deep vein thrombosis – DVT).

The following are some of the more common side effects of gastric band surgery.

• Infection in the region of your gastric band, the tube under your skin, or in one of your wounds. If this happens, your skin can become red and tender.

• During surgery, you may damage your stomach or other surrounding organs like your liver or spleen.

• Your gastric band can come loose, leak and deflate, or gradually work its way through your stomach wall. The band would need to be repositioned, removed, or replaced if any of these occur.

• If you lose weight too quickly, you may develop gallstones. These can be painful, and removing them can necessitate surgery.

If you experience any symptoms after your surgery, such as a fever, stomach pain, chest pain, breathlessness, or constant vomiting, call your doctor or surgeon.

Not everyone loses as much weight as they want to after the operation, and some people gain weight after losing it. If this occurs, your surgeon can prescribe alternative treatments such as gastric bypass surgery.

Chapter 4: WHAT IS EMOTIONAL EATING

What is emotional eating?

A common but unhealthy way to cope with difficult feelings or emotions can be emotional eating. When you are upset or stressed, or rely on food as a treat or reward for a tough week, to motivate yourself, or even as a fallback when you are bored, if you find yourself reaching for food, these can all be signs that you are using food to help boost your mood. This can lead to feelings of guilt, shame, and even a cycle of unhealthy eating habits over time that can lead to problems with eating, disordered eating, and physical health issues.

A hypnotherapist can use hypnosis to encourage you to recall long-forgotten experiences surrounding food that may now subconsciously affect you. They will also help you identify patterns, responses, or habits that you do not know you have been doing. Before beginning gastric band hypnotherapy, discussing and identifying any unhealthy thinking patterns concerning food may be beneficial.

Next, the virtual gastric band treatment will be carried out by your hypnotherapist. Gastric band hypnotherapy is intended to indicate that you have undergone an operation to implant a gastric band at a subconscious level. The intention is for your body to respond to this suggestion by making you feel fuller faster than having the actual surgery.

In contrast to diets, getting a virtual gastric band is designed to help you make big changes in your lifestyle. Hypnotherapy can help you take those first steps towards making positive change by recognizing and addressing underlying issues, helping you to recognize triggers, and working with your subconscious to help you feel fuller for longer.

Diets do not seem to cope with the necessary lasting changes in lifestyle, such as a positive long-term shift in eating habits and food attitude. Many diet plans are temporary, often because they are too restrictive, or they completely deprive us of our favorite foods and can be difficult to maintain on an ongoing basis.

These regimes can be adhered to in the short term, but they do not work well in the long run. Many diets can make us more obsessed with food and eating by causing us to count calories or consciously measure portion size, or even totally omit food types. This can take the pleasure of eating out and leading us to want more certain foods and begin a diet-overeat/binge cycle.

Unhealthy relationships with food

It may also be worth considering your relationship with food if you consider weight-related surgery or hypnotherapy alternatives. Simply focusing on the ultimate goal of weight loss can often overlook the underlying problems of an unhealthy relationship with food that can affect you in various areas of your life, including affecting your self-confidence, self-esteem, causing feelings of anxiety or guilt, or even holding you back in social or work-related situations.

The eating problem does not have a single look.' It can affect anyone in any number of different ways, at any age. It's important to talk with your GP if you're worried that your eating habits may affect your overall health and well-being.

EMOTIONAL EATING AND HOW TO STOP IT

Do you eat or relieve stress to feel better? These tips can help you stop emotional eating, combat cravings, recognize your triggers, and find more satisfying ways to feed your emotions.
What is emotional nutrition?

Just to satisfy physical hunger, we don't always eat. For comfort, stress relief, or to reward ourselves, many of us also turn to food. And we tend to reach out for junk food, candy, and other comforting but unhealthy foods when we do. When you feel down, you might reach for a pint of ice cream, order a pizza if you are bored or lonely, or swing by the drive-through after a stressful day at work.

Emotional eating uses food to make yourself feel better than your stomach, to satisfy emotional needs. Emotional eating, unfortunately, doesn't fix emotional issues. It generally makes you feel worse. Afterward, the original emotional problem not only remains, but you feel guilty for overeating as well.

- Are you an emotional eater?
- When you are feeling stressed, do you eat more?
- When you are not hungry or when you are full, do you eat?
- Do you eat to feel better (when you're sad, crazy, bored, nervous, etc.) to relax and soothe yourself?
- Are you rewarding yourself with food?
- Do you eat regularly before you have yourself stuffed?
- Does food make you feel protected? Do you have the feeling that food is a friend?
- Do you feel powerless around food or out of control?

The cycle of emotional eating

It isn't necessarily bad to occasionally use food as a pick-me-up, a reward, or celebration. But when eating is your primary emotional coping mechanism, you get stuck in an unhealthy cycle where the real feeling or problem is never addressed, when your first impulse is to open the refrigerator whenever you are stressed, upset, angry, lonely, exhausted, or bored.

With food, emotional hunger can't be filled. Eating may feel good at the moment, but there are still the feelings that triggered the eating. And due to the unnecessary calories, you have just consumed, you often feel worse than you did before. For messing up and not having more willpower, you beat yourself.

You stop learning healthier ways to cope with your feelings, you have a harder and harder time controlling your weight, and you feel increasingly powerless about both food and your emotions, compounding the issue. But it is possible to make a positive change no matter how powerless you feel over food and your feelings. You can learn to deal with your emotions in healthier ways, avoid triggers, conquer cravings, and finally stop emotional eating.

The distinction between hunger for emotions and physical hunger

You first need to learn how to distinguish between emotional and physical hunger before you can break free from the cycle of emotional eating. This can be trickier than it sounds, especially if you use food to deal with your feelings regularly. Emotional hunger can be strong, so it's easy to mistake physical hunger for that. But to help you tell physical and emotional hunger apart, there are clues you can look for.

Suddenly, emotional hunger emerges. In an instant, it hits you and feels overwhelming and urgent. Physical hunger, on the other hand, happens more slowly. The urge to eat does not feel as dire or demand instant satisfaction (unless you haven't eaten for a very long time).

Emotional hunger craves particular foods for comfort. Almost anything sounds good when you're physically hungry, including healthy things like vegetables. Emotional hunger, however, craves junk food or sugary snacks that provide an immediate rush. You feel like you need a cheesecake or pizza, and you're not going to do anything else.

Emotional hunger often results in eating mindlessly. You've eaten a whole bag of chips or an entire pint of ice cream before you know it, without really paying attention or enjoying it fully. You're usually more conscious of what you're doing when you feed in response to physical hunger.

Emotional hunger until you're full isn't satisfied. More and more, you keep wanting, always consuming until you are uncomfortably stuffed. On the other hand, physical hunger does not require stuffing. When your stomach's full, you feel satisfied.

Emotional malnutrition is not in the stomach. You sense your hunger as a craving that you can't get out of your mind, instead of a growling belly or a pang in your stomach. Specific textures, tastes, and smells are what you concentrate on. Sometimes, emotional hunger contributes to remorse, shame, or disgrace. You are unlikely to feel guilty or embarrassed when you eat to relieve physical hunger since you are giving your body what it wants. It's probably because you know deep down that you're not eating for nutritional purposes if you feel bad after you feed.

Emotional hunger comes on suddenly	Physical hunger comes on gradually
Emotional hunger feels like it needs to be satisfied instantly	Physical hunger can wait
Emotional hunger craves specific comfort foods	Physical hunger is open to options — lots of things sound good
Emotional hunger isn't satisfied with a full stomach.	Physical hunger stops when you're full
Emotional eating triggers feelings of guilt, powerlessness, and shame	Eating to satisfy physical hunger doesn't make you feel bad about yourself

Identify the reasons for emotional eating

Identifying your causes is the first step in putting a stop to emotional food. What circumstances, locations, or emotions make you reach for the comfort of food? Most emotional eating is related to negative feelings, but positive emotions, such as thanking yourself for completing a goal or enjoying a holiday or happy event, may also cause it.

Popular emotional eating triggers

Uh, stress. Do you ever notice how stress makes you starve? This isn't just in your head. Your body generates high levels of the stress hormone cortisol when stress is chronic, as it is so often in our stressful, fast-paced world. Cortisol induces cravings for salty, sweet, and fried foods that provide you with a burst of energy and enjoyment. For emotional relief, the more uncontrolled tension in your life, the more likely you are to resort to food.

Emotion Stuffing. Eating may be a way to silence or 'stuff down' negative feelings temporarily, like frustration, anxiety, depression anxiety, isolation, resentment, and shame. When you're numbing yourself with food, the difficult feelings you'd rather not feel can be stopped.

Boredom or lonely thoughts. Do you ever eat either to give yourself something to do, reduce boredom, or fill your life with a void? You feel unfulfilled and hollow, and your mouth and your time are consumed by food. It fills you up at the moment and distracts you from your life's underlying feelings of purposelessness and disappointment.

Habits for infancy. Think back to memories of your childhood with food. Did your parents reward good behavior with ice cream, take you out for pizza when you received a good report card, or serve your candy when you felt sad? Such trends may also carry on into adulthood. Or your eating can be inspired by nostalgia for cherished memories of grilling burgers with your father in the backyard or baking and eating cookies with your wife.

Influences from social. A perfect way to alleviate stress is to get together with other people for a meal, but it can also lead to overeating. It's easy to overindulge simply because the food is there or because someone else is feeding. You might even overeat out of nervousness in social settings. Or maybe you're motivated to overeat by your family or circle of friends, and it's easier to go along with the party.

Keep an emotional eating diary

In at least a couple of the previous examples, you have probably recognized yourself. But you'll want to get even more precise, even so. One of the easiest ways to describe the trends behind your emotional eating is to keep track through a diet and mood journal.

Take a moment every time you overeat or feel tempted to reach for your version of Kryptonite comfort food to find out what induced the impulse. Usually, if you backtrack, you can discover a disturbing incident that began the emotional eating cycle. In your food and mood log, write it all down: what you ate (or wanted to eat), what happened to bother you, how you felt before you ate, what you felt when you ate, and how you felt afterward.

You'll see a trend emerge over time. Perhaps you still end up gorging yourself with a vital friend after spending time. Or even if you're on a deadline or when you attend family events, you stress feeding. The next step is to find healthy ways to feed your emotions once you identify your emotional eating causes.

Try other ways of feeding your emotions

You will not be able to control your eating habits for too long if you don't know how to handle your emotions in a way that doesn't include food. Diets too often fail because they provide logical dietary guidance that only works if the eating habits are actively managed. When emotions hijack the process, expecting an immediate reward with food, it doesn't work.

To prevent emotional eating, you have to find other ways to relieve yourself mentally. It's not enough to understand the emotional eating cycle or even understand your causes, even though it's a big first move. For emotional satisfaction, you need alternatives to food that you can turn to.

Alternatives to emotional eating

Call anyone that always makes you feel better if you're sad or lonely, play with your dog or cat, or look at a favorite picture or favorite memento.

Expand your nervous energy by dancing to your favorite tune, holding a stress ball, or taking a brisk walk if you are anxious.

Give yourself a hot cup of tea if you're tired, take a bath, light some scented candles or cover yourself in a warm blanket.

Read a good book, watch a comedy show, explore the outdoors, or turn to an activity you love when you're bored (woodworking, playing the guitar, shooting hoops, scrapbooking, etc.).

Stop and check in with yourself when cravings strike and About their food cravings, most emotional eaters feel helpless. It's everything you can think about when the desire to eat strikes. Right now, you sense almost crippling stress that needs nourishment! Since you tried and failed to resist in the past, you conclude that your willpower is just not up to snuff. The reality, however, is that you have more control than you realize over your cravings.

Take five before you give in to a craving

Emotional eating appears to be essentially senseless and automatic. You have reached for a bowl of ice cream and polished off half of it before you even know what you are doing. But if you can stop and think for a moment when you're stuck with an urge, you give yourself the chance to make a different choice.

Is it five minutes you can put off eating? Or just one minute to start with. Don't tell yourself that you can't give in to craving; note, incredibly tempting is the forbidden one. Tell yourself just to wait.

Check-in on your own while you're waiting. How do you feel? What's happening emotionally? You'll have a better idea of why you did so, even though you end up eating it. This will help you set yourself up next time for a different answer.

Learn to accept your feelings — even the bad ones

Although the central issue may seem to be that you're powerless over food, emotional eating simply stems from feeling powerless over your feelings. You don't feel capable of coping head-on with your emotions, so with food, you stop them.

It can be frightening to allow yourself to sense unpleasant emotions. You may be afraid that, like Pandora's box, you won't be able to shut it once you open the door. But the fact is that even the most unpleasant and challenging feelings relatively easily subside and lose their power to dominate our attention when we don't obsess over or block our emotions. You need to become aware and learn how to remain connected to your emotional experience from moment to moment to do this. This will help you to rein in stress and fix emotional issues that sometimes trigger emotional eating.

Indulge without overeating by savoring your food

You prefer to do it easily, mindlessly eating food on autopilot when you eat to feed your emotions. You eat so quickly that you miss the various tastes and textures of your meal, as well as the signs that your body is full and not hungry anymore. So you will not only enjoy your food more by slowing down and savoring each bite, but you will also be less likely to overeat.

A significant element of mindful eating is slowing down and savoring your food, the opposite of mindless, emotional eating. Before beginning your meal, try to take a few deep breaths, put your utensils down between bites, and just concentrate on the eating experience. Pay attention to your food's textures, shapes, colors, and smells. What does each mouthful taste like? How does your body feel about it?

You'll find you enjoy each bite of food much more by slowing down in this way. You can also indulge in your favorite foods and feel a lot less loaded. It takes time to enter your brain with the body's fullness signal, so taking a few moments to remember how you feel after each bite, hungry or fulfilled, will help you stop overeating.

Practice mindful eating

Eating when you are also doing other things will keep you from completely enjoying your meal, such as watching TV, driving, or playing with your phone. Since your mind is elsewhere, even if you're no longer hungry, you can not feel full or continue eating. Eating more carefully will help concentrate your mind on your diet and the enjoyment of overeating and curbing a meal.

Support yourself with good habits for lifestyle

You're better able to navigate the curveballs that life eventually throws your way when you're physically strong, relaxed, and well-rested. But any little hiccup can take you off the rails and straight to the refrigerator when you're already tired and stressed. Without emotional eating, exercise, sleep, and other good lifestyle behaviors can help you get tough times.

Making routine workouts a priority. Physical exercise does wonders for your mood and energy levels, and it's also a strong reducer of stress. And it is easier than you may think to get into the exercise habit.

Every night, strive for 8 hours of sleep. Your body craves sugary foods that will give you a fast energy boost if you don't get the sleep you need. Having plenty of rest can help with appetite regulation and decrease cravings for food.

Allow time for relaxation. Give yourself permission to relax, decompress, and unwind each day for at least 30 minutes. This is your chance to take a break and refresh your battery from your duties.

• Communicate with others. Don't underestimate the value of social activities and close relationships. It will help shield you from the negative effects of stress by spending time with positive people who enrich your life.

5 STRATEGIES TO HELP YOU STOP EMOTIONAL EATING

Don't let feelings cause poor eating habits
You're standing in the freezer, steaming over your wife's war, looking for some ice cream to calm your emotions. After a long day, you sit on the couch and mindlessly munch through a whole bag of chips.
This is to feed emotionally. "You may have heard it called "stress eating," but "emotional" is more appropriate, says Anna Kippen, MS, RDN, LD, a registered dietitian. Many negative emotions may cause poor eating habits, including rage, depression, and stress.

Here's the issue: In fact, the feel-good foods you reach for can make you feel worse. Fortunately, there are techniques to help ensure that your emotions do not turn into diet harm in the long term.
1. Get down to the underlying cause
Short-term concerns include a rough day at work or a fight with a friend. But emotional eating can also result from broader problems. These include chronic stress, frustration, depression, and other issues over the long term. You can benefit from therapy, stress management, exercise, and other techniques if these apply to you.
The tactics outlined here will assist. But finally, you need to recognize the underlying cause of your emotional eating and fix it.
2. Ask why you eat

When you go to the freezer, pantry, or vending machine, take a break and ask yourself a simple question: "Am I really hungry?" "

On a scale of 1 to 5, Kippen recommends ranking your appetite, with one being that you're not hungry at all and five being that you're so hungry that you're going to consume the food you hate the most in the world.

"Just diving into mindless eating is too easy, but by asking yourself this question, you at least acknowledge your motivation," she says.

She recommends taking a healthy, balanced snack within 15 minutes or a healthy, balanced meal within 30 minutes if your appetite clocks in at level three or four. If your physical appetite is lower than that, she suggests that you pursue an alternative activity, such as drinking a cup of fruity herbal tea or taking a stroll.

"She says, "Becoming more conscious of your level of hunger will help you curb unnecessary snacking and make better decisions.

3. Swap out the worst of your snacks

You can't eat the whole bag if you don't have a huge bag of greasy chips at your fingertips. That's good since overeating processed snacks can increase the levels of the stress hormone cortisol.

Suppose you need a salty snack, stock up on popcorn (only with salt and oil). You'll get all of the grains that are an essential source of serotonin, the feel-good hormone. You'll also get antioxidants and far fewer calories than chips to improve the immune system. Another excellent crunchy choice with protein and fiber is roasted chickpeas to fill you up.

If your sweet tooth is caused by tension, rage or disappointment, note this: The sugar high comes afterward with a low. This decrease will contribute to increased cravings later on. Certain emotional concerns, including signs of depression, can also worsen with candy and processed foods.

Kippen suggests holding a bowl of sweet fruit out in the open as an alternative to your favorite sweets, cake, or pies. (Studies show that you're more likely to eat fruits and veggies).

She says, "I also suggest keeping frozen berries on hand that can be thrown into a blender quickly to make a healthy sorbet."

4. Choose foods that fight stress

Have you ever wondered why, in emotional circumstances, people give hot tea? There's more to it, it turns out than calming steam. Tea also includes beneficial antioxidants. And there is an amino acid called L-theanine in green tea, matcha tea, and white tea that can help reduce stress levels.

Try dark cherries if you happen to have snacks late at night. They not only deliver a tasty treat but also help increase your natural melatonin levels to help you sleep. Similarly, salmon and other omega-3 fatty acid-rich fish can help with sleep. Dark chocolate (at least 72% cacao), whole grains, nuts, legumes, and fruits and vegetables all play a role in keeping a balanced mind. The list goes on. Kippen says, "The key is to stock up on foods that help with your stress or emotions and to avoid processed junk that could make you feel worse."

5. Make emergency packages

If you're susceptible to snacking due to stress, plan for it. Don't eat any food straight from the box, for example. Grabbing snacks is a recipe for binge eating and overindulgence from the box.

Instead, in baggies or cans, pre-portion treats like almonds, popcorn, or sliced veggies. Find these, or just your balanced snack choices on an ongoing basis, your emergency snack packets.

Beyond these tips, it should be repeated: Ask for it if you need medical support to fix emotional problems. With a full treatment plan, a doctor will help you handle stress, depression, frustration, or other negative emotions.

What to expect: getting a gastric virtual band

An initial consultation will likely be your first meeting with the hypnotherapist to discuss what you hope to gain from hypnotherapy. This is a chance to talk about any previous attempts at weight loss, your eating habits, any health problems, and your general food attitude. This data will give the therapist a clearer idea of what will help and whether any other forms of treatment should be taken into account or not. Note: it's important to seek advice from your doctor if you have any health problems relating to your weight.

The procedure itself is designed to imitate the gastric band's surgery to assist your subconscious in believing that it happened. Many hypnotherapists will incorporate the sounds and smell of an operating theatre to make the experience more authentic. By taking you into a deeply relaxed state, also known as hypnosis, your therapist will begin. At all times, you will be aware of what is happening and will be in control.

The therapist will talk you through the operation once you are in a hypnotic state. From being put under the anesthetic to making the first incision, fitting the band itself, and stitching up the cut, they will explain step by step what happens in surgery. To convince your subconscious that what is being said is happening to you, the sounds and smells of an operating theatre will improve the experience.

During the process, other ideas may be implemented to improve self-confidence. Your hypnotherapist can teach you some self-hypnosis techniques once the treatment is complete to help you stay on track at home.

Some hypnotherapists may recommend returning for follow-up appointments to help track the virtual gastric band's performance and make any changes. This occurs as individuals also mount the physical band. For others, as part of a long-term weight-loss strategy, maintaining hypnotherapy sessions may be helpful. This encourages the hypnotherapist to work with you to fix the underlying diet and self-esteem problems.

Hypnosis of the gastric band should form part of a weight management program that addresses nutrition and exercise habits. It is the combination of changing habits in both the body and mind that is often most successful for those seeking weight loss.

How am I going to feel afterward?

For those who over-eat, it can be hard to recognize when you're physically full. Sometimes we eat, ignoring whether or not we are physically hungry, purely for taste or comfort. To cultivate healthy eating habits, learning to recognize the physical sensations of being hungry and full is helpful.

With most individuals reporting a calm feeling when they come out of hypnosis, the procedure should be a pleasant and relaxing experience.

Will hypnotherapy for the gastric band work for me?

For those attempting hypnotherapy for the first time, a common question is: will it work for me? Sadly, it's not a simple case of yes or no; it's largely up to you. Hypnotherapy helps people with a range of concerns, but it is especially useful when it comes to changing habits. It is often successful, for this reason, in helping people develop healthy eating habits and lose weight. However, just like any other lifestyle change, it will require your total commitment.

No method of weight loss is guaranteed to achieve specific outcomes, from surgery to diets. Similarly, gastric band hypnotherapy results, as with any form of hypnosis, depend on you approaching the process with an open mind and being ready and willing to make changes.

If you trust in the process and your therapist, you are more likely to make sustainable modifications and get what you want from gastric band hypnotherapy. It is important to be relaxed and trust your hypnotherapist. This is why it is recommended that you take time in your field to study hypnotherapists and find out more about them, how they function, and what their qualifications include. Before you begin, you should arrange to meet with them to guarantee that you feel comfortable with them.

Gastric band hypnosis should work for you if you are dedicated to making a lifestyle change, believing in the process, and trusting your hypnotherapist.

Is a gastric virtual band the right solution for me?

It can depend on many different factors if a virtual gastric band is right for you or not. It can be a great alternative to traditional surgery for some individuals. Others may find it a useful instrument for creating positive lifestyles and sustainable weight loss. It's important to remember that there are many different solutions and options available to you, whatever your situation is.

Chapter 5: LOSING WEIGHT

Losing weight can be a difficult process - not made any easier
by the conflicting advice out there in the world and often
dangerous. With TV programs, advertising, and social media
feed full of food photos, we are constantly bombarded. The
presence of these can make the temptation to move away from
healthy or intuitive eating very strong.

Then there are pills for weight loss and other commercial
weight reduction programs that focus on limiting what you
eat rather than considering how you eat or what you think
about the food you put into your body. It is no surprise that
some negative mindsets have developed around what we put
in our bodies.

Weight loss hypnosis can be an effective way to challenge
these mental attitudes and temptation moments, helping you
live a healthier life.

The goal of weight loss hypnotherapy is to make you feel
confident about your body, change negative eating thoughts,
and help you responsibly lose weight without affecting your
emotional well-being. A hypnotherapist can help you develop
a positive relationship with food and exercise, which is key to
healthy weight loss and long-term weight management, by
targeting the unconscious mind with powerful suggestion
techniques.

Is it necessary for me to lose weight?

Many people insist that, whether they are overweight or not,
they need to lose weight. But the truth is, very few
individuals, regardless of whether they need to lose weight,
are happy with the shape and size of their bodies.

Body confidence

While individuals need to lose weight if they are overweight for health reasons, it's not good to feel ashamed of the need or desire to lose weight. Since body shape and size are so linked to the western concept of beauty, people are constantly searching for quick fixes' to cut corners.

Some of the ways people attempt to lose weight are weight loss supplements, fad diets, and grueling workout regimes. What you need to ask yourself is - am I happy to do this? For the rest of my life, can I continue doing this?

This is where weight loss hypnotherapy can improve. You need to first change your mind to change your body. Why am I dissatisfied with my body, and why can't I lose weight? You must ask yourself.

How does hypnosis for weight loss work?

Hypnotherapy for weight loss is becoming more common, and it is good for maintaining a healthy weight in the long term for people all over the world.

Over time, you will learn how to substitute your negative habits and to eat behaviors with healthy ones recommended by your hypnotherapist - and a series of weight loss hypnotherapy sessions.

What occurs during weight loss hypnosis?

Your hypnotherapist will direct you into a state of deep relaxation.

Your hypnotherapist will be able to reach your unconscious mind until your body and mind are completely relaxed (the part of us that operates all the time but that we are not aware of, i.e., instincts and survival mechanisms).

It is possible to use relaxing, carefully worded scripts to discuss why a client overeats and proposes new ways of thinking through visualizations. Without any input from your hypnotherapist, you have the power to ignore any suggestions you don't feel comfortable with. For some of the strategies and visualizations they can use, see below.

- Hypnotherapy for techniques to lose weight

- While each scenario is different and everyone has their reasons for wanting to lose weight, some suggestions that you might encounter include:
- Imagining the body you want or the fitness/health level you want to attain.
- Imagining how your new look and health will make you feel.
- Imagining yourself comfortably hitting that target.
- Seeing how far from today you would have changed.
- Imagine how energized and secure you will feel.
- Realizing that the more you workout, the more you will want to exercise and the easier it will become to do so.

These techniques are designed to empower you so that you can take control of your choices. If you're worried that your relationship with certain types of food is becoming unhealthy, hypnotherapy for food addiction could help you break these negative thought patterns.

You can learn to love the taste of healthy food by weight loss hypnosis and avoid craving sugary, fatty foods. You should also learn not to see it as a source of anxiety but to love your body. Hypnosis for weight loss can help you adopt a healthier lifestyle and a happier mindset by tackling those deep feelings that form the foundations of your eating habits.

Your possible weight loss blocks

For a variety of reasons, plenty of individuals attempt and struggle to lose weight. These causes are mostly unconscious, otherwise referred to as 'secondary benefits,' making it impossible for us to resolve them.

It is worth looking at the confidence that has held the weight in place for so long when someone loses weight. We always hold beliefs at two levels; we think positive thoughts about ourselves, our worth, and what we deserve as human beings at the conscious level; but our habits unconsciously give away our emotional beliefs.

Amreeta Chapman/Aujayeb, a clinical hypnotherapist, discusses the issues people can face while losing weight.

The fact is, by not making changes, we can sometimes gain security - we feel comfortable remaining just as we are. So, we may want to consciously lose weight, but something in the subconscious keeps us from making it a reality. Weight loss hypnotherapy seeks to uncover these causes, helping consumers to eventually push through obstacles that could have stopped them from losing weight for several years.

How to overcome secondary gains and lose weight with hypnosis is explored in the following video.

We'll take a look below at some of the reasons you may find it difficult to lose weight successfully.

You eat comfort from food

We learn to equate feeding with the warmth of our mothers when we are infants. Some experts believe that this association never really leaves us, so we can return to those early days of total dependence when life gets stressful. This is where it can become an issue for emotional eating.

If you have ever found yourself after a long day reaching for a chocolate bar, or ordering a takeaway when you feel lonely and sad, then you could be a comfort eater. You will find it harder to lose weight as a comfort eater because you have let food become your coping mechanism and, without it, you do not know how to cope with your emotions.

Hypnotherapy will help fix this, allowing you to understand how negative feelings are handled in a way that does not contribute to eating comfort.

The biggest change is that I have been much less bothered to eat. I love it, but when my body is hungry, I have learned to feed, not only because my mind needs anything to soothe my feelings.

You're eating mindlessly,

You have to be fully frank about how much you eat and exercise to lose weight. It's easy to forget about the occasional snack here and there, even though you keep a food diary or use a food-tracking app. Maybe when you make dinner, you choose the ingredients? Do you catch something on your commute to work, or do you tuck your afternoon tea into a biscuit?

These 'on the go' foods always catch us out; however, they always add up. Even if you religiously stick to salad for dinner, it won't do you any favors to conveniently ignore all the things you eat in between. This sort of mindless eating is something weight loss hypnotherapy can help you to resolve. If you struggle with conscious feeding, gastric band hypnotherapy might help you. The idea is to make you feel fuller for longer, which may help stop excessive day-long grazing.

You're banning food

Like a mystery package you're told not to open, it can make them all the more desirable by removing those foods from your diet. If you find yourself limiting the foods you consume, when your willpower takes a dip, you're more likely to want to binge.

Learning to eat attentively is the secret to sustainable and effective weight loss. You'll be able to enjoy your favorite foods in moderation and stop piling on weight if you can eat carefully, savoring every bite.

A key part of weight loss hypnosis is helping customers eat consciously - putting aside emotional factors and developing a stable relationship with food that promotes a long-term, healthy weight.

You don't exercise enough

When it comes to weight loss, exercise is just as relevant as diet. Sometimes mental blocks can stop us from wanting to exercise, including:

Feeling an absence of energy

Feeling too self-conscious to publicly exercise

Convincing yourself that you're going to go tomorrow' (every day)

Hypnotherapy for weight loss will help you break down the mental blocks that stop you from making the most of your body. Having your body working and your heart pumping more often than not can help you feel better about yourself in general, contributing in the long run to healthy habits and satisfaction.

Will hypnosis for weight loss work for me?

One of the most frequently asked questions in hypnotherapy sessions is - can weight loss hypnotherapy function for me? The response to that is, before you try it yourself, it's hard to tell. While it definitely won't work the same way for everyone, when it comes to diet and exercise, the process of talking about creating healthy habits and getting rid of poor habits can help build a new level of knowledge.

Hypnotherapy is supportive treatment, a vital point to remember, and can also be used with a balanced eating and exercise routine. You can find it helpful to talk to your doctor or nutrition professional if you want advice about eating healthy and exercising. Of all these aspects, it is always a combined effort that contributes to results.

5 Reasons Many Diets Fail (and How To Succeed)

For every diet that they go on, the average person gains 11 pounds. Perhaps worse, they lose muscle and fat as they lose weight. They get all the fat back as they regain the weight. And because muscle burns seven times as many calories as fat, their metabolism is slower than when the diet began. The cruel reality is that to maintain their weight, they then require even fewer calories.

Didn't you know someone who was overweight and told you that they didn't eat that much? Maybe they aren't lying. They just damaged their metabolism through dieting with a yo-yo.

Two simple things are the key to losing weight and holding it off. First, not by white-knuckling it and starving yourself, but by fixing the out-of-whack hormones and brain chemistry that drive hunger and over-eating, you automatically reduce your appetite.

The second is to automatically increase your metabolism, so you burn more calories all day long. Unfortunately, most diets do the opposite – increase hunger and slow metabolism.

Here are the five reasons most diets fail and how to succeed.

1. To control your appetite, you use willpower instead of science.

The science of hunger is there. Sadly, most diets can cause hunger (eating less). Only for so long can you hold your breath. For so long, you can just starve yourself. Powerful ancient mechanisms make up for and protect us from hunger (even if it is self-induced). Our appetite increases significantly, our cravings ramp up, and our metabolism slows down to conserve energy. It increases appetite and reduces metabolism by consuming certain foods (low fat, higher carb, or sugar foods).

The Principle of success: Appetite

Enough food to satisfy your appetite (but only real whole fresh food).

For breakfast, consume protein and stop eating 3 hours before bed.

To regulate blood sugar and lower insulin, write your meals. At each meal, combine protein, fat, and low glycemic, non-starchy carbohydrates (vegetables, fruit, small quantities (less than half a cup of grain and beans). Insulin spikes are delayed by fat, protein, and fiber.

2. You're focusing on calories (eating less and exercising more)

The calorie in/calorie out mantra of energy balance as the secret to weight loss is entering the scientific dustbin fast. In my last Automatic Weight Loss article, I reviewed the science behind the reality that not all calories are made equally.

Some calories make you fat; they make you slim with some calories. We now know that a change in your metabolism is caused by any food that spikes insulin (sugar, flour, and even excess grains, fruit, and beans). What's insulin doing? It pushes all the fuel in your blood into your hungry fat cells from the food you just ate (visceral or belly fat).

Then your body thinks you're starving, even though it's just a huge bagel or a large gulp swallowing you down. And note, when your body feels you're starving, two things happen—you increase appetite and slow metabolism.

Did you ever eat a big meal, and then, an hour later, did you feel hungry again, and you had to go raid the fridge or eat something sweet? That's the explanation.

Success Principles: Calories

Focus on very low-glycemic foods as the diet's staples. Nuts, seeds, chicken, pork, meat-fed on turf, low glycemic vegetables (greens, salad fixings, etc.)

Sparingly use the grains and beans

Use sugar, in very small doses, as a medicine. And sugar is just the same. "If you have to ask the question "is OK? "It's not. They trigger sweet receptors, appetite, and sluggish metabolism, leading to obesity and type 2 diabetes. Do not use artificial sweeteners.

3. You eat a low-fat diet

Most people also believe we can stop egg yolks and help them lose weight by consuming a low-fat diet. The old principle that fat has nine calories per gram and carbs have four calories per gram contributed to the misguided belief that we will lose weight if we cut out fat.

Yeah, look what's happened to America in the last 30 years, where the rage and weight loss tool has been low fat. We are fatter than ever (70% of us are overweight), and now there is pre-diabetes or type 2 diabetes or what I like to call "diabesity" in 1 in 2 Americans.

Walter Willet, a Harvard scientist, reviewed all the science on low fat and weight loss and discovered that eating fat is not what makes you fat, but sugar. David Jenkins' recent study found that a low-carb (26 percent), high-fat (43 percent) vegan diet was more effective than a low-fat vegan diet for weight loss and reducing cardiovascular risk factors. The high-fat party lost four more pounds by eating high fat and lowered their cholesterol by ten more points. It was called Eco-Atkins! Other studies indicate that you can increase your metabolism by 300 calories a day by eating more fat and fewer carbs (eating the same total calories a day). That is like having the advantage of running without getting off the sofa for an hour a day. Sit on your ass and lose 1 pound every 11 days. You might call it "The Butt Diet."

Success Principles: Fat

• Don't worry about fat. It makes you feel complete, accelerates your metabolism, and helps you lose weight.

At each meal, eat good fat.

Eat vegetable fats, such as avocado, nuts, coconut butter, seeds, or oil,

Eat clean animal fats (yolk, chicken, grass-fed organic eggs) and fish with omega-3 fats (sardines, herring, wild salmon, black cod).

4. You have concealed reasons and need medical assistance

Beyond your diet or amount of exercise, some reasons influence your weight and metabolism. Your body is a system, and it affects the metabolism of many things. In my books, The Blood Sugar Solution or The Blood Sugar Solution 10-Day Detox Diet, I've written about them.

The things that cause inflammation are the largest hidden causes of weight gain or weight loss resistance. And inflammation from anything that, by worsening insulin resistance, causes weight gain.

What triggers inflammation?

Hidden allergies to or food sensitivities. Gluten and dairy are the most common culprits. But do not turn to alternatives that are gluten-free or dairy-free. Gluten-free cakes and biscuits are still pastries and biscuits. In sugar and refined carbs and flours, they are still very strong. With the sweeteners, just try soy yogurt. You're not going to eat it!

Gut Problems. The microbiome plays a major role in metabolism and health—the 100 trillion bacteria in your gut. If you have bad bugs, they can either cause inflammation or alter how your food is broken down and consumed (eating processed, high-sugar, carb, low-fiber diets or taking antibiotics, acid blockers). The metabolism of fecal transplants from a lean person to an obese person would change. And what is next? Poop transplants for weight loss. Probably!

Toxins. Science has discovered that common environmental chemicals (pesticides, household cleaners, make-up, pollution, and heavy metals) can be "obesogens." Chemicals that make you fat. In animal studies, giving toxins to rats caused weight gain even if they consumed and exercised the same amount of calories.

Success Principles: Find Hidden Causes of Weight Gain

Try a diet for elimination. Not cutting calories, just getting rid of inflammatory foods. Get started with gluten and milk. For three weeks, 100 percent.

• Patch the stomach. Stop medications that are gut-busting (acid blockers, antibiotics, and anti-inflammatories). Eating a low-glycemic, low-fermentation (starch) diet starves the bad bugs. Grab probiotics. If you don't work on your own, see a specialist of Functional Medicine get help.

Detox your physique and your life. Reduce exposure to chemicals that are environmental and normal. See the Environmental Working Group tools to minimize exposure to skincare ingredients, household products, and foods you consume (meat and veggies). And a resource from the NRDC for consuming fish without mercury. Eat 2 cups a day of cruciferous veggies (broccoli family). To conduct a medically supervised detoxification program, you may need help from a Functional Medicine doctor.

5. You haven't got a plan.

Health isn't something that's happening to you, either. You have to schedule something, like a holiday or your retirement! Most of us fail because we are not "designing our health." We are not setting up automatic performance conditions.

One of the days in my book, The 10-Day Detox Diet, focuses on the "Design" concept. How do you design your life so that you do not have to worry about doing the right thing? Have all the right foods in the house, the right ingredients all ready for your morning protein shake, create an emergency travel food pack, have your week-long exercise plan. You create conditions to make it easy.

Also, we find that doing things together makes it easier for them. We got 15,000 individuals at Saddleback Church to lose 250,000 pounds in a year by having them do it together. Every corpse needs a friend! It makes it fun and makes it work to join groups of individuals doing this in person or an online community or group. To redesign their lives for good, we have created online challenges where people have had profound success.

Find out what works for you; just don't expect to be safe. You've got to plan on it!

Success Principles:

- Create a Plan
- Commit your health to design. Do it on Sundays every week!
- Create an emergency food package for life.

- Join a community or have a friend or a buddy.

Chapter 6: ALL YOU NEED TO KNOW ABOUT WEIGHT LOSS HYPNOSIS

Hypnosis may be best known as the party trick used to make people on stage do the chicken dance, but more and more people turn to the technique of mind control to help them make healthier choices and lose weight. Case in point: The dieting veteran turned to hypnosis when Georgia, 28, decided she needed to lose the 30 or so pounds she had put on after foot surgery in 2009. In the past, the mind-control technique had helped her overcome a fear of flying, and she hoped that it would also help her create healthy eating habits.

The self-proclaimed foodie was initially surprised by the advice of her hypnotherapist. Eat when you're hungry, listen to your body and eat what you want, stop when you're full, eat slowly and enjoy every mouthful,"[She had] four simple agreements to which I would need to adhere: Eat when you're hungry, listen to your body and eat what you crave, stop when you're full, eat slowly and enjoy every mouthful,"[She had] four simple agreements that I would have to adhere to: "As such, no foods were off-limits, and I was encouraged to eat everything in moderation-music to my ears!"

Who Should Try Hypnosis

For anyone seeking a gentle way to lose weight and make healthy eating a habit, hypnosis is for everyone. One person that this isn't for? Everybody was interested in a quick fix. It takes time to reframe problematic ideas about food - Georgia tells her hypnotherapist eight times a year, and it took a month before she began to notice a real change.

"The weight dropped off slowly and surely, without huge changes to my lifestyle. I was still eating out numerous times a week, but often sending plates back with food on them! For the first time, I was tasting my food, spending time to take in flavors and textures. Almost ironically, it was as if I had recommenced my love affair with food; only I was able to lose weight doing so," she said.

How to Use Hypnosis to Lose Weight

Traci Stein, Ph.D., MPH, an ASCH-certified health psychologist in clinical hypnosis and the former Director of Integrative Medicine in the Department of Surgery at Columbia University, says that hypnosis is not meant to be a "diet" but rather a tool to help you succeed in eating nutritious food and exercise. "Hypnosis helps people experience in a multi-sensory way what it feels like when they are strong, fit and in control and to overcome their mental barriers to achieving those goals," she says. Hypnosis can specifically help people resolve the underlying psychological problems causing them to hate exercise, experience intense cravings, binge at night, or eat mindlessly. It helps them identify the triggers and disarm them."

It's helpful not to think of hypnosis as a diet at all, says the certified hypnotherapist at the Houston Hypnosis Center, Joshua E. Syna, MA, LCDC.

"It works because it changes their way of thinking about food and eating, and it allows them to learn to be more calm and relaxed in their lives. So instead of food and eating is an emotional solution, it becomes an appropriate solution to hunger, and new patterns of behavior are developed that enable the person to deal with emotions and life," he explains. "Hypnosis works for weight loss because it enables the person to separate food and to eat from their emotional life."

Dr. Stein says it is fine for people with no other mental health concerns to use at-home self-guided audio programs created by a certified hypnotist (look for an ASCH certification). But beware of all the new online apps - one study found that most apps are untested and often make grandiose claims that can not be substantiated about their effectiveness.

What Feels Like Hypnosis

Forget about what you've seen in movies and on stage; therapeutic hypnosis is closer than a circus trick to a therapy session. "Hypnosis is a collaborative experience, and the patient should be well-informed and comfortable every step of the way," Dr. Stein says. And for people who are worried about being tricked into doing something odd or harmful, she adds that if you don't want to do something, even under hypnosis, you won't. "It's just focused attention, "It is just focused attention. "Everyone naturally goes into light trance states several times a day - think of when you zone out while a friend is sharing every detail of their vacation - and hypnosis is just learning to focus that inward attention helpfully." Dispelling from the patient's side the myth that hypnosis feels weird or scary, Georgia says she always felt very lucid and under control. There were also amusing moments where she was told to imagine walking on the scale and seeing her target weight. "My overly creative mind had to first imagine myself removing all clothes, every bit of jewelry, my watch, and hair clip before jumping on in the nude. Anyone else does that, or is it just me?" (No, it's not just Georgia!)

THE ONE DOWNSIDE OF WEIGHT LOSS HYPNOSIS

It is non-invasive, works well with other therapies for weight loss, and needs no tablets, powders, or other supplements. Nothing happens at worst; putting it in the "might help, can't hurt" camp. But Dr. Stein admits that there is one drawback: the price. Costs per hour vary depending on your location, but for therapeutic hypnosis treatments, it ranges from $100-250 dollars an hour, and when you see the therapist once a week or more for a month or two, which can add up quickly. And hypnosis isn't covered by most insurance companies. Dr. Stein, however, notes that it could be protected if it is used as part of a broader mental health treatment package, so consult with the provider.

A Surprising Perk of Hypnosis Weight Loss

Peter LePort, MD, a bariatric surgeon and medical director of the MemorialCare Center for Obesity in California, says that hypnosis is not only a mental thing but also a medical component. "You must deal with any underlying metabolic or biological causes of weight gain first, but while you're doing that, using hypnosis can kickstart healthy habits," he says. And the use of hypnosis is another healthy advantage: "The meditation aspect can help reduce stress and increase mindfulness which in turn can help with weight loss," he adds.

So, does hypnosis work for weight loss?

A surprising amount of scientific research looks at the efficacy of weight loss hypnosis, and much of it is positive. One of the original studies conducted in 1986 found that, compared to 0.5 pounds for women who were just told to watch what they ate, overweight women who used a hypnosis program lost 17 pounds. In the '90s, a meta-analysis of hypnosis weight loss study found that subjects who used hypnosis lost more than twice as much weight as those who didn't. And a study in 2014 found that hypnosis women improved their weight, BMI, eating behavior, and even certain body image aspects.

But it's not all good news: a Stanford study in 2012 found that about a quarter of people simply can't be hypnotized, and it has nothing to do with their personalities, contrary to popular belief. Rather, the brains of some people just do not seem to work that way. "If you're not prone to daydreaming, often find it hard to get engrossed in a book or sit through a movie, and don't consider yourself creative, then you may be one of the people for whom hypnosis doesn't work well," Dr. Stein says.

One of the success stories is certainly Georgia. It not only helped her shed the extra pounds, she says, but also helped her hold them safe. Six years later, although she needed a refresher, she happily continued her weight loss, sometimes checking back in with her hypnotherapist.

What Is Weight Loss Hypnosis and Does It Work?

You already know about the usual go-to professionals regarding losing weight: doctors, nutritionists, and dietitians, personal trainers, even mental health coaches. But there might be one that you haven't talked of quite yet: a hypnotist.

Using hypnosis, it turns out, is another road people venture down in the name of weight loss. And typically, after all the other last-ditch attempts (I see you, juice cleanses and fad diets) are tried and failed, it's traveled, says Greg Gurniak, a certified Ontario clinical and medical hypnotist.

But it's not about someone else controlling your mind while you're unconscious and making you do funny things. "The biggest misconceptions about hypnosis are mind control and loss of control, aka doing something against your will," says Kimberly Friedmutter, hypnotherapist and author of Subconscious Power: Use your inner mind to create the life you've always wanted. "People are relieved to see I'm not wearing a black robe and swinging a watch from a chain because of how the entertainment industry portrays hypnotists."

When you experience hypnosis, you're also not unconscious; it's more like a deep state of relaxation, explains Friedmutter. "Before you drift off to sleep, it's simply the natural, floating feeling you get or that dreamy feeling you feel as you wake up in the morning before you are fully aware of where you are and what is around you."

Being in that state makes you more prone to change, and that's why weight loss hypnosis may be effective. "It differs from other techniques because hypnosis directly addresses the cause and other contributing factors in the mind of the person at the subconscious level, where their memories, habits, fears, food associations, negative self-talk, and self-esteem germinate," says Capri Cruz, Ph.D., psychotherapist and hypnotherapist and author of Maximize Your Super Powers. "No other method of weight loss addresses the core problems at the root as hypnosis does."

But does hypnosis for weight loss work?

There is not much recent, randomized research available on the topic, but what is out there indicates that the technique could be plausible. Early studies in the 1990s found that people who used hypnosis lost more than twice as much weight without cognitive therapy as those who died. A 2014 study worked with 60 obese women and found that those who practiced hypnobehavioral therapy lost weight and improved their eating habits and body image. And a small 2017 study worked with eight obese adults and three children, all of whom lost weight successfully, with one even avoiding surgery because of the benefits of treatment, but none of that is conclusive, of course.

"The unfortunate factor is that hypnosis is not readily covered by medical insurance, so there isn't the same push for hypnosis studies as there is for pharmaceutical ones," Dr. Cruz says. But with the seemingly ever-increasing cost of prescription drugs, long lists of possible side effects, and the push for more natural alternatives, Cruz is hopeful that as a plausible approach to weight loss, hypnosis will soon receive more attention and research.

For weight loss, who should try hypnosis?

Anyone who has trouble sticking to a healthy diet and exercise program is, honestly, the ideal candidate because they can not seem to shake their negative habits, Gurniak says. It is a sign of a subconscious problem to get stuck in harmful habits, like eating the entire bag of potato chips instead of stopping when you're full, he says.

Your subconscious, Friedmutter says, is where your feelings, habits, and addictions are located. And it may be more effective because hypnotherapy addresses the subconscious rather than just the conscious. In reality, a 1970 study analysis found that hypnosis had a success rate of 93 percent, with fewer sessions needed than both psychotherapy and behavioral therapy. "This led researchers to believe that hypnosis was the most effective technique for changing habits, thought patterns, and behavior," Friedmutter says.

Hypnotherapy also doesn't need to be used on its own. Gurniak says that hypnosis can also be used as a complement to other programs designed by professionals to treat different health conditions, such as diabetes, obesity, arthritis, or cardiovascular disease, for weight loss.

During treatment, what can I expect?

Depending on the practitioner, sessions can vary in length and methodology. For instance, Dr. Cruz says her sessions usually last between 45 and 60 minutes, whereas Friedmutter sees patients with weight loss for three to four hours. But in general, with your eyes closed, you can expect to lay down, relax and let the hypnotherapist guide you through specific techniques and suggestions that can help you achieve your objectives.

"Friedmutter says, "The idea is to train the mind to move towards what is healthy and away from what is unhealthy. I can determine subconscious hitches through client history that have sent the client away from their original [health] blueprint. We should learn to respect them just as we learn to abuse our bodies with food.

And no, you're not going to cluck like a chicken or confess any profound, dark secrets. "Gurniak says, "You can not be stuck in hypnosis or made to say or do something against your will. "If it goes against your values or beliefs, during the trance, you will simply not act on the information given."

Instead, Gurniak adds, you will likely experience deep relaxation while still being conscious of what is being said. Someone would describe it as being between being wide awake and asleep in a hypnotic trance," he says." They are fully in control and able to stop the process at any moment because if you choose to, you can only be hypnotized. We work as a team to achieve the objective of the individual.

Of course, depending on your response to hypnosis, the number of sessions needed is completely dependent. Others might see results in as little as one to three, Dr. Cruz says, while others would require eight to 15 sessions somewhere. And then again, for everyone, it can not be successful.

5 BENEFITS OF HYPNOTHERAPY WEIGHT LOSS

It can prove difficult to achieve the ideal weight, especially for people who have tried various techniques, including exercise regimes and dieting. When you are unable to lose weight, it can be very upsetting, affecting your self-confidence and self-esteem. This can adversely impact your relationships and job. Hypnosis for weight loss is a perfect technique if you feel you've run out of options or want to try something new. Here are the weight-loss advantages of hypnosis.

Increased trust

Increased faith can be gained by individuals taking part in hypnosis. This can be seen as people start meeting their targets for weight loss. You will start feeling better about yourself with several hypnotic sessions. Furthermore, in a new light, you will also see yourself, and this will give you the much-needed boost in your confidence.

More energetic resources

Hypnosis for weight loss can also help you to improve your energy levels. Your energy levels will rise as you start reducing your body weight. To keep you active and happy, this increased energy is ideal. It will also motivate you with both family and friends to do something that you love. You would no longer have to deal with low levels of energy that are typically related to obesity.

Increased span of life

Studies have shown that their life expectancy rises by several years when individuals lose healthy weight. Hypnotic weight loss helps you maintain your perfect weight, which helps you live a happier and fulfilled life. You will also get some of your life back as you begin to see the effects of your hypnosis therapy. Easywillpower.com has all the information about the hypnotic weight loss treatment that you need.

Deal with psychological issues

Psychological problems can lead individuals to engage in unhealthy behaviors that, over time, can increase their weight. There are individuals, for instance, who find comfort in food when they are stressed. Hypnosis therapy may help to sever the link between eating and the emotional turmoil that exists. This implies that they will only eat food when they are hungry, not when they feel stressed. Therefore, depending on food as their source of comfort, they will stop.

Help lose weight for you

Weight loss hypnosis can unconsciously help people to reinforce beneficial eating habits. Hypnosis can allow people to develop healthier lifestyles because they will naturally come to your body and mind with all good habits. Studies have shown that people who have received hypnotic therapy lose more weight than 90% of those who have not received hypnosis. Also, hypnosis will help keep the weight off for the long-term.

Reduce stress

Patients can be less stressed and more mindful of the act of going into a trance. Less stress is important because greater productivity and increased trust will be guaranteed.

Awareness will help to identify the various impulses and will also assist you in taking care of your food cravings.

It can be difficult to lose bodyweight, particularly when you have to stick to a consistent schedule that includes exercise and dietary restrictions. A variety of medically supervised services, including surgery, pharmacotherapy, pre-packed meals, and behavioral improvements, may be selected. Hypnotherapy is also an alternative technique for weight loss that works perfectly for most individuals, especially when other conventional attempts fail.

Chapter 7: HYPNOSIS VS MEDITATION: THE DIFFERENCES EXPLAINED

Meditation by Hypnosis VS is a duel without a clear winner. Hypnosis and meditation seem similar, and to keep their stress, anxiety, and depression in check, millions of individuals worldwide rely on these practices. But at first, glance, although the practices seem similar, there are significant differences between the two.

We take a closer look at hypnosis and meditation in the following article, and we examine the differences between them.

HYPNOSIS

what is hypnosis? According to the American Psychological Association, there are many definitions you could use, but hypnosis is a cooperative interaction between a responsive participant and a suggestive hypnotist.

Hypnosis became well-known thanks to popular acts and Hollywood movies, although it is a clinically proven practice, where people are encouraged to act ridiculously and behave like chickens.

Hypnosis provides medical and therapeutic advantages, despite its image in modern media, and it is particularly effective in treating pain and anxiety. Hypnosis can decrease the symptoms of dementia or other mental illnesses, some studies suggest.

How Hypnosis Functions

For over 200 years now, scientists have disputed hypnosis, and science has yet to explain everything in the hypnotized brain. We can detect when a person's brain is activated under hypnosis; thanks to modern technology such as fMRIs, we can see the exact moment when a person enters hypnosis, but we can't clearly explain why the person does it.

But we have a good understanding of hypnosis's general features, even though some details are missing, and we can predict its effects. Hypnosis is a trance state that is distinguished by extreme suggestibility, increased imagination, and mind and body relaxation.

Hypnosis is compared with sleep by many individuals, but the two mental states are not alike. A hypnotized one is alert at all times, unlike a sleeping person. It would resemble a state of daydreaming or the feeling you get when your mind is 'lost' in a good book or movie to compare hypnosis with something. You are aware of what's going on around you, but all but the subject you're focusing on, you can tune out.

During the hypnosis session, everything you experience seems somewhat real to you, much like something that happens in a book or movie seems real. The incidents fully engage your feelings. Depending on what you're watching or reading, you feel sad, happy, or fearful. Well, the hypnotist guides your mind during a guided hypnosis session, so you can face your fears, tackle your sadness, or embrace your happiness.

Some researchers consider forms of self-hypnosis to be daydreaming and immersive experiences while reading or watching movies. A psychiatrist who specialized in hypnosis, Milton Erickson, believed that people were hypnotizing themselves daily. He said that psychiatrists have the distinct advantage of knowing how to induce a state of relaxation that makes a trance state possible and guide the mind towards useful topics by using focusing exercises.

To begin making beneficial and brilliant changes in your life, check out all of Mark's hypnosis downloads that can be accessed today.

The State of the Hypnotic

When we move from wakefulness to sleep, deep hypnosis is often described as a state of relaxation similar to what we experience. During conventional hypnosis sessions, as if they were real, you approach your ideas or the ideas that your hypnotist suggests.

You might feel a tingling sensation in your hand and have trouble closing your fist if the hypnotist were to suggest that your hand was swollen. You might feel a cooling sensation in your mouth if the therapist suggests that you eat ice cream. If the hypnotist suggests that you are facing something you fear, you might begin to sweat and increase your heart rate. But you should know that all that's going on is inside your head. Your mind is pretending to play. If the hypnotist proposed that you behave like a chicken, you would be conscious that it is not in your interest, and you would not comply with it. Relaxation and a lack of inhibitions define the hypnotic state. Most researchers say this happens because without letting our concerns, worries, and suspicions interfere with our actions, we can concentrate on something. We focus on the storyline while watching a movie we enjoy, and our worries and suspicions melt away. When we're in a hypnotic state, the same thing occurs, but instead of concentrating on a movie story, we concentrate on ourselves.

People, when they are in a hypnotic state, are highly suggestible. That's why most people would consider the hypnotist's advice and adopt it as their own. The fear of humiliation disappears, and you open up to the moment. But you are still conscious of your environment, so you can't be convinced by the hypnotist to do something you don't like.

MEDITATION

What Is Meditation?
Meditation is defined as a collection of methods designed to inspire an improved state of mental awareness and concentrated attention.

In almost every faith, including Buddhism, Judaism, Islam, Christianity, and Hinduism, meditative practices are found. Even though meditation is mostly used for religious reasons, without having any spiritual or religious inclinations, many people practice it.

Meditation is an important psychotherapeutic method. Simple procedures such as listening to our breath, repeating a mantra, or detaching our thinking process allow us to concentrate our attention on a particular subject. Furthermore, these procedures trigger a state of self-awareness and inner relaxation that can enable us to hone our concentration. Meditation shows us that while we can not control certain aspects of life, we can control our states and adjust them for the better. With the help of meditation, we learn that we can overcome our personal sorrows, fears, anxieties, and confusions with the help of our minds.

Now, how about attempting this guided meditation?

How Meditation Functions

Meditation can take many forms, but we can group them into two key types: a meditation on mindfulness and concentrative meditation.

Meditation on mindfulness targets anxiety and depression, but it may also concentrate on other subjects. Mindfulness meditation requires being conscious of and engaged in the present moment and making yourself aware of your life's continuing course, and embracing it.

When blocking out everything around us, Concentrative meditation teaches us to concentrate our attention on particular objects. Whether it's our breath, a mantra, or a flower, the purpose of this form of meditation is to completely experience what we're concentrating on. Experiencing stuff with our whole being enables us to achieve a greater state of being.

THE MEDITATIVE STATE

The place of meditation is relaxed without making you slouch. Most individuals who have been meditating for a while suggest it's easy to enter a meditative state. Well, once you get the knack of it, it is simple. Most of us will need to practice and learn how to meditate, even though some people have no trouble entering a meditative state.

We can enter a meditative state, some of the most popular advice states, if:

We get into a position where we do not feel pain, but we are also not comfortable. And if you think about the popular role of meditation in modern media that we see, you get it. The role is not awkward, but it also doesn't encourage you to recline or to sleep.

Closing our eyes and tracking our respiration. It can take us a couple of minutes to reach a meditative state. Slowly but surely, concentrating all our energy on breathing in and out will lower our breathing rate. This process will not only keep our minds focused, but it will also lower our heartbeat and relax the body.

We can start some mental exercises once our breathing is heavy, such as concentrating on our hands, feet, and back. We should note how they feel and push any distractions away.

Scientists have not worked out exactly how and why it functions, even though meditation has many therapeutic and health benefits. Meditation works because it alters the strength of our brain waves, one theory suggests.

There are five categories of brain waves:

1. The Gamma State (30-100 Hz) is the first one. This is the condition that our brain enters when it is learning actively or when it's hyperactive. The Gamma state is great for keeping data, and it's one of the reasons why good educators connect and switch around so often

with their audiences. The teachers improve the chances of long-term assimilation of the data by keeping our minds stimulated. In the Gamma state, our brains can't function for a long time because it's tiring. Overstimulation also contributes to anxiety that can prevent the data from being assimilated by our brains.

2. The Beta State (13 to 30 Hz) is the second type of brainwave. This is the emotional state of the day that most of us have. The beta state is connected to 'thinking' or 'working' and helps us prepare and analyze our world.

3. The Alpha State (9 – 13 Hz) is the third brainwave. A slowing down of the thought mind characterizes this state. We feel calm and relaxed when this state is involved. This is the brain state most of us have after pleasurable sexual experiences or after a stroll in the woods or other stimulating activities. This brain state causes lucid but analytical thought and a slightly diffused perception.

4. The Theta State (4 – 8 Hz) is the fourth brainwave. When we enter this mental state, we begin meditation. This is where the brain switches from a meditative and visual state to a verbal and thought mode. Slowly, the planning mind drifts away and makes room for a deeper state of consciousness and a stronger problem-solving capability.

5. The Delta State (1 - 3 Hz) is the fifth and last form of brain waves. This mental state can be reached by will by Tibetan monks who have been meditating for most of their lives, but most of us can only reach it while sleeping.

6. Meditation can help us switch from one type of brainwave to another by lowering our breathing and heart rates and relaxing our minds and bodies. We can

hit the fourth brain wave with practice, and some may even reach the fifth with enough practice. Consistency is crucial when it comes to meditation. Shorter meditation sessions are more effective at regular intervals than longer sessions that are unevenly spaced.

WHY PEOPLE ASSOCIATE HYPNOSIS AND MEDITATION

The hypnotherapist and the meditation guide do different things
1. The Hypnotist And The Guide to Meditation
The rising popularity of guided meditation is one of the reasons people associate hypnosis and meditation. People turn to guided meditation because, without learning how to meditate, it enables them to tap into meditation's benefits. It's a faster process, and it is preferred over others by many. By offering descriptive instructions, the meditation guide, a trained practitioner, leads one or more people through meditation.

The meditation guide may be mistakenly associated with a hypnotist by some. They have nothing in common besides the fact that both professionals use verbal instructions to guide their customers through their process.

Licensed physicians and psychologists use hypnotherapy to treat multiple conditions and mental illnesses. Certified hypnotherapists assist individuals in managing their weight and give up smoking and help them cope with addiction.

Meditation guides or teachers help people reach a meditative state, but they do not have the training to overcome their fears or give up smoking by helping their trainees. The clients have an increased awareness once they achieve a meditative state and can reach the same conclusions on their own, but the processes vary greatly.

To help the client reach the hypnotic state and concentrate on their problems, the hypnotist uses well-placed suggestions. At the same time, the meditation guide depends on the ability of the client to enter the meditative state.

2. The Hypnotic State And The Meditative State

While at first, they might appear identical, the hypnotic and the meditative states are distinct. Both require you to be conscious of your environment, but this is where things vary. Your mind is aware of everything when you are in a hypnotic state, but it focuses on the hypnotist's suggestions. You will have a sharp focus with the help of these suggestions, and you will address the matters you want to resolve, whether you want to quit smoking or sleep better.

On the other hand, your mind is also aware of everything when you're in a meditative state, but you focus on your breath, on your hands and feet, or an object. This will increase your self-awareness and may shed new light on your issues, but it will not be highly effective in quickly treating a particular condition.

3. Both Topics Are Shrouded In Myths

Hypnosis and meditation are both shrouded in legends.

Yet another reason that many individuals confuse hypnosis and meditation is that myths are shrouded in both. In modern media, both topics have been falsely or negatively depicted. People still think hypnotists will make them dance like chickens on the stage and that meditation is something that ninjas do to hone their senses.

These stereotypes do not help anyone, and these stereotypes are fostered by the presence of self-entitled specialists who do not know what they do on shows.

The reality is that the people you see acting like chickens on stage are paid actors who allow themselves to engage in these stupid displays.

The truth is, ninjas may have been meditating, but they haven't done it to hone their senses. They were meditating, just as modern people do, to increase their awareness and calm their nerves.

People still think meditation makes levitate monks. We will not discuss the possibility of levitation, but if you start meditating, the chances of lifting over the ground are inexistent.

People often fear that they will not remember anything from their hypnosis session or surrender their will to the hypnotist and risk dominating them.

The truth is that hypnosis can cause amnesia, but it's a good thing that rarely happens. They might lose their grip on reality when people enter a deep hypnotic trance. But even though this may sound scary, entering a deep into a trance would require most people's long-term memory, so the suggestions of the hypnotist will have a powerful effect.

It is nothing but a myth to surrender your will and do what the hypnotist wants you to. During a hypnosis session, you're still mindful of yourself, and hypnotherapists are nothing like the showmen you see on stage. It's not possible to force hypnosis on others. It's something people do for themselves. As a facilitator, a hypnotherapist serves, and he or she will guide you to achieve your goals and nothing more.

HYPNOSIS VS MEDITATION: WHY THEY DIFFER
Hypnosis and meditation help your mind to overcome different issues
Hypnosis and meditation vary, but they are identical as well. Both processes help your mind face and overcome different problems and provide health and therapeutic benefits.

Hypnosis and meditation are different, despite their similarities, and they are achieved in different ways. Hypnosis can help you accurately treat various conditions, while meditation can help you become a better person.

I am sure you have a clear idea after reading this article about which process might be more beneficial for your particular problems.

Chapter 8: FOOD ADDICTION AND HOW TO OVERCOME IT

Some people find it difficult to avoid certain foods because of their effects on the brain.

Food addiction works in the same way as other addictions, which explains why certain people can not control themselves around specific foods, no matter how hard they try.

Despite not wanting to, they may find themselves consuming large quantities of unhealthy foods despite knowing that doing so may harm them.

This chapter looks at food addiction and offers strategies for overcoming it.

What is food addiction?

Food addiction is an addiction to junk food and comparable to drug addiction.

It's a recent — and contentious — term, and reliable statistics on its prevalence are lacking.

Food addiction is similar to several other disorders, including bulimia, compulsive overeating, binge eating disorder, and other eating and feeding disorders.

Effects on the brain

Food addiction involves the same regions of the brain as drug addiction. Furthermore, the same neurotransmitters are involved, and many of the symptoms are the same.

Processed junk foods have a profound effect on the brain's reward centres. These effects are triggered by brain neurotransmitters like dopamine.

Typical snack foods, such as candy, sugary soda, and high-fat fried foods, are among the most problematic foods.

Food addiction is thought to be triggered by a dopamine signal that activates the biochemistry of the brain, rather than a lack of willpower.

Eight symptoms of food addiction
Food addiction cannot be diagnosed with a blood test. It is focused on behavioral symptoms, much like other addictions. Here are 8 common symptoms:

1. Constant cravings for specific foods, despite feeling full and having just finished a healthy meal,
2. Starting to eat a craved food and end up consuming more than you intended
3. Eating a craved food and sometimes eating to the point of feeling excessively stuffed
4. Feeling bad after consuming those foods, then eating them again shortly afterward
5. Make excuses on why it's a good idea to give in to a food craving
6. Repeatedly — but unsuccessfully — attempting to stop consuming such foods or establishing rules on when it is permissible to consume them, such as at cheat meals or on specific days.
7. Many people hide their unhealthy food intake from others.
8. You are feeling unable to stop yourself from eating unhealthy foods, despite knowing that they damage your health or cause weight gain.

If you have more than four or five of the symptoms on this list, it could indicate a serious issue. If you answered yes to six or more of the questions, you most likely have a food addiction.
Though the word "addiction" is often used casually, having a true addiction is a serious disorder that almost always requires treatment.

Food addiction shares many of the same symptoms and thought patterns as drug addiction. It's just a different substance, and the social implications may be relatively mild. Food addiction can affect one's health and lead to chronic illnesses such as obesity and type 2 diabetes.

Furthermore, it can have a negative effect on a person's self-esteem and self-image, causing them to be dissatisfied with their image.

Food addiction, like other addictions, can be emotionally draining and increase a person's risk of dying young.

How to know whether avoiding junk food is worth the sacrifice

It can seem difficult to stay away from junk food entirely. They're everywhere, and they're a big part of today's culture. However, in some cases, completely avoiding certain trigger foods may be necessary.

Once you've made the firm decision never to eat them again, avoiding these foods can become simpler as the need to justify eating — or not eating. Cravings can also go away or become noticeably less intense.

Consider making a list of advantages and disadvantages to help you think through your decisions.

• Advantages. These may include living longer, having more energy, losing weight, and feeling better every day.

• Disadvantages. These may include not eating ice cream with relatives, not being able to bake cookies during the holidays, and trying to explain food choices.

Write everything down, no matter how vain or peculiar it may seem. After that, compare the two lists and decide if it's worth it.

If the response is a resounding "yes," be rest assured that you've made the right choice.

Also, bear in mind that many of the social problems that might appear on the list can be easily resolved.

First steps in overcoming food addiction

There are a few things that will help you prepare for giving up junk food and make the transition smoother:

- Trigger foods. Make a list of the foods that cause your cravings and/or binges. These are the cause foods to avoid absolutely.
- Fast food places. Make a list of fast food places that serve healthy foods and take note of their healthy options. This may help you avoid relapsing when you're hungry and don't feel like cooking.
- What to eat. Consider what foods to consume, ideally nutritious foods that you like and eat regularly.
- Pros and cons. Make several copies of the pro-and-con list. Make copies and keep them in your kitchen, glove box, and purse or wallet.

Additionally, do not go on a diet. Put weight loss on hold for at least one to three months.

Overcoming food addiction is tough enough. Adding hunger and restrictions to the mix would certainly make it more difficult.

After taking these preparatory steps, set a date in the near future — like the coming weekend — on which the addictive trigger foods will not be touched again.

Consider seeking help

Most addicts try to quit several times before finally succeeding in the long run.

Although it is possible to conquer addiction without assistance — even if it takes many attempts — it is often helpful to seek assistance.

Many support groups and Many health professionals and can aid in overcoming your addiction.

Finding a psychiatrist or psychologist with experience dealing with food addiction may offer one-on-one support, but some free group options are available.

These include 12-step programs like GreySheeters Anonymous (GSA), Food Addicts Anonymous (FAA), Overeaters Anonymous (OA), and Food Addicts in Recovery Anonymous (FA).

These groups meet on a regular basis — some even via video chat — and can provide the necessary support to help people overcome their addictions.

Food addiction is an issue that does not usually go away on its own. Unless you make a deliberate effort to deal with it, chances are it will get worse over time.

The first steps toward overcoming the addiction is to list the benefits and drawbacks of stopping trigger foods, find healthier food alternatives, and set a date to begin the journey toward health.

Consider seeing a health professional or joining a free support group. Keep in mind that you are not alone.

Chapter 9: SELF ESTEEM, INSECURITY, AND OBESITY

The voice of insecurity and self-doubt can be persistent, loud, discouraging, and even detrimental to our efforts. We've all experienced toxic self-talk in various aspects of our lives. The importance of self-esteem in achieving life goals, such as weight loss, cannot be overstated. It is a factor in all our human endeavors. Understanding how our self-esteem has been affected and influenced throughout our lives will help us in gaining the necessary awareness to effective change.

It Begins at Birth

The feedback and comments begin as soon as the baby is born, with phrases like "Oh, what a lovely baby!" "What a big baby!" Of course, the baby is completely unconcerned. However, before long in life, the child realizes the importance of the feedback they get from the world around them. Praise and criticism are ingrained in our psyches and are difficult to forget, particularly if they are negative.

We develop self-esteem as we realize how necessary it is to begin to fulfill the standards of others. We start looking for clues to our worth, acceptability, and identity in others. We may often conceal our true selves inside and focus all of our attention on satisfying others. Our self-esteem is shaped by the feedback we get from the world around us and how we perceive it. People make comments about others on personality, weight, appearance, looks, or talent, which can be complimentary or unfavorable.

Psychological Cravings

Humans have two psychological cravings. The first is for love, warmth, affection, and care. Children desperately want to be loved. That is what provides a sense of security to a child and an adult. Kids believe that there is one place where they will always be loved: their "home." Most parents make an attempt to satiate this hunger on a regular basis. The craving follows us into adulthood, though it is no longer as "needy."

The second craving humans have is for recognition, approval, or affirmation. Kids aren't shy about it, "Mom, look what I got in school today;" "Dad, are you coming to my soccer game?" . This is what shapes and molds our sense of self-worth. This hunger for approval is carried from the family into society. As we get older, the cravings do not go away, but they are nourished in different ways. And sometimes, as adults, we have to satisfy our cravings. Compliments are never too plentiful in society, especially in the workplace.

As the child grows older and attends daycare, starts school, visits relatives and peers, maintains relationships, attends church, joins clubs, participates in sports, and later in life gets a job and begins working on a career, criticism and comments will come, often uninvited. Our self-esteem is shaped and influenced by this feedback.

Awareness of Feedback

We become more aware of feedback such as reactions, looks, comments, avoidance, the occasion of being ignored, not being picked for the squad, the engagement in conversation, doing well or poorly in school, evaluations at work, winning and losing competitions, interactions with neighbors and friends, and assessment of career goals. We all hope for positive feedback.

However, we all know there would be negative feedback: the one comment a parent, teacher, or relative made that can always reverberate in our minds, such as a friend's unexplainable rejection, a coach who placed a label to us, a peer who was blatant in his or her dislike, comments on our size or weight, etc.

The more positive feedback we get and internalize, the more confident we feel in ourselves. The more negative reviews we get, the more insecure we become. We will begin to build a barrier around ourselves to shield ourselves from excessive scrutiny, shaming, labeling, or any other adult-scripted failure in our lives.

Making the journey back into our developmental history of self-esteem and asking ourselves what feedback did people, especially significant others, offer us about our personality, intellect, friendliness, appearance, looks, life potential, creativity, lack of talent, behavior, and our body is a useful reflective activity.

Dealing with Comments

We have no control over others' uninvited comments, but we do have control over how we react to them. We're all familiar with society's negative responses to obesity, and when it's personalized, it can be devastating. Teasing, critiques, looks, rejections, exclusions, accusations, and phrases have all been mentioned by many patients over the years. It can be painful, regardless of how well we defend ourselves.

The pain may be concealed, subdued, or ignored, but it is still there, weakening our sense of security. We may have also agreed with the negative feedback and embraced it as part of our identity, whether consciously or unconsciously.

Suggestions to Help

- Give yourself the right to feel good about yourself and more secure: say out loud to yourself when no one else is present, "I have the right to feel good about myself." It's necessary to hear yourself say these words out loud for them to be effective. You may need to repeat it many times to match the feelings to the words. The more you repeat the sentences, the more they will become ingrained in your mind.

- If you were brainwashed as a child that you didn't have the right to feel good about yourself, you might need to give yourself "permission" to do so: "I want to give myself permission to feel good about myself." Repeat it until you believe it.

- Choose a few affirmation statements to incorporate into your positive thinking. Some statements inspire you to change your negative self-talk in ways that matter to you. For example, "I affirm my intelligence." "I affirm my ability to be good in what I want to do."
- Write a few affirmation sentences specific to you on your mirror and repeat them aloud every morning and during the day until they become part of you.
- Counseling and life coaching will assist you in fostering positive self-perceptions that influence our self-esteem.

We will be more effective in achieving any behavioral goal if we have a secure and confident "self." As children, we couldn't "fight back" but as adults, we can affirm ourselves, program positive thoughts into our minds, silence the negative "voices" in our heads, choose not to be influenced by comments, filter feedback and encourage self-confidence.

You will rehabilitate a shattered and insecure sense of self-worth. The goal is to re-program negative thoughts in your mind and replace them with positive ones over time, as this isn't an overnight process. Let me encourage you to build a strong sense of self-worth over time and use it to achieve your weight-loss goals.

Chapter 10: HOW TO BE CONFIDENT AS A OVERWEIGHT ADULT

In the United States, 70.7 percent of adults over the age of 20 are considered overweight. However, as an overweight adult, you might occasionally feel alone or self-conscious about your appearance. Fortunately, you can develop self-confidence and strive for a healthy and happier relationship with your body, which can lead to a more satisfying life. You can learn to be more positive about yourself by concentrating on body positivity, addressing negative thoughts and low self-esteem, and seeking inspirational figures.

Building Confidence in Your Body

1. Remind yourself of the great stuff your body can do. It can become easy to concentrate on what you can not do. Rather than concentrating on them, think about a few incredible things you might do, such as singing, painting, and playing an instrument.

- Some people find it beneficial to consider also the basic functions of their bodies. For instance, "My body is strong enough to carry me throughout the day."

2. Dress in clothes that make you feel good about yourself and your body. When choosing your outfit, try not to be concerned about what other people should think or say about it. Choose clothing that reflects your personality and compliments your figure.

- For example, if you like a specific TV show, see if you can find a shirt in your size that features a character or phrase from the show on Etsy or RedBubble.
- Choose your best features and purchase clothing that accentuates them. Wear high-waisted trousers and boots to elongate your thighs if you're taller and have longer legs.
- If you're not sure what to wear to flatter your figure, consider following some "guidelines" for dressing in figure-flattering clothes. Ask for advice at a shop that caters to plus-size bodies. You should dress well and look put-together regardless of your size.
- Don't be concerned about the size on your clothing label. These are just numbers; they don't describe you! You are a unique person who is more than just a number on the label.

3. A trip to the spa or a day of rest will pamper your body. Taking care of your body is sometimes the only thing you can do for it! Make an appointment at your nearest spa for a facial or massage, or take a soothing bath at home. Take advantage of this opportunity to pamper yourself and take care of your skin, muscles, and hair. Take a bath, give yourself a manicure and pedicure, exfoliate and moisturize your skin, and apply an at-home facemask to create your own mini spa day at home.

4. Be critical of ads that tell you how you're supposed to look.

Unfortunately, there are many businesses that profit from people's insecurities. When you see ads for clothing or weight loss items, think about whether the company wants you to feel bad for yourself and buy their product to make you feel better. If a company claims that their product would make you more attractive or appropriate, they are most likely preying on your insecurities.

- For example, if an advertisement begins with the phrase "Want to get rid of those unsightly fat rolls on your stomach and back?" the purpose of the advertisement is to make you self-conscious about something that most people experience regardless of their weight. The advertisement conveys the impression that fat rolls are unsightly and undesirable. You're more likely to be interested in what they're offering if you're self-conscious about your appearance. Advertising aims to make you feel a certain way in order to elicit an answer to a product or brand. In most cases, companies want you to purchase a product. It's easier to fight the urge to feel bad about your body if you understand what they're doing in their advertisements.
- Pick up a magazine that uses normal-sized models instead of magazines that try to make you feel bad! More brands are beginning to use real people as models instead of unrealistic, photo-shopped pictures.
- Pay attention to the body's cues on what it needs. Trusting your body is a big step toward self-assurance. Become aware of whether you're hungry, thirsty, energized, or tired, and try to meet your body's needs at that time. Try to live your life based on what your body is telling you it wants rather than what other people or ads are telling you.
- Living this way will also contribute to a healthy overall lifestyle. It may take some practice, but with dedication, it is entirely possible.

- It's important to remember that you and your doctor should talk about your health and weight. If your doctor believes that your weight is affecting your health, work with them and develop a strategy for living a healthy lifestyle.

Combating Low Self-Esteem

1. Work toward goals you've set for yourself. Follow your dreams! Make a list of your goals, and break them down into small, measurable steps. Check in with yourself on a daily basis to see how far you've come! If you are working for something important to you, you will have less time to think about your weight.

- Setting health-related goals, such as increasing your activity level or consuming more vegetables, is a good idea. However, make sure you're still pursuing your life goals, such as getting a degree, landing a dream job, extending your artistic life, hosting an open mic night, or starting your own herb garden.

2. Remind yourself that you have the right to be happy with who you are. Giving yourself permission to feel good will help when you're struggling with a lack of confidence. Stand in front of a mirror and practice saying , "I have the right to feel good about myself and my body." You can also construct a mantra that makes you feel good and reminds you of your worth.

- If you're having trouble with negative thoughts about your body, try redirecting them into positive ones by saying something like, "It is okay to feel bad sometimes, but I know I am a beautiful person inside and out."

- Even though you don't believe what you're saying right now, simply repeating the word will make you feel better.

3. See a therapist to talk about any negative feelings or behaviors. Make an appointment with a therapist if you constantly feel sad or even depressed as a result of your weight. Talk to them about your relationship with your body and why you feel down on yourself. A therapist will also assist you in developing a strategy for improving your behavior.

- Your therapist can also assist you in overcoming cognitive distortion, which is a common problem. You may have a tendency to exaggerate what's going on in your life, such as by having all or nothing thinking, jumping to conclusions, trying to read other people's minds, only seeing the negative in a situation, or assuming other people's behaviors are because of you. Your therapist will help you identify when this occurs so that you can learn how to stop.

- Keep in mind that the therapist is there to assist you, not to punish or shame you for your negative feelings.

- If you can't afford therapy, go to a counseling clinic at a local university that offers a mental health counseling program. They occasionally offer free or heavily discounted sessions to help Sometimes, To assist graduate students in gaining patient experience.

4. Surround yourself with self-assured and encouraging people. Make friends with outgoing, kind, polite, and upbeat people. Search for "body positive" groups in your area, to meet other people who have struggled with low self-esteem or a negative self-image, . Do not be afraid to cut ties with those who make you feel bad about yourself because of your appearance or weight.

- Speak up when your mates say body-negative things about themselves and others. If anyone says something derogatory about their body, say something like, "You're a beautiful person inside and out!" . Let's concentrate on what we like about ourselves rather than what we don't."

5. Compliment yourself and others for qualities other than appearance. Low self-esteem can result from putting too much emphasis on how you look. Shift your frame of reference by praising other people and yourself for skills and qualities that are not related to looks. This will help you recognize your own value while also encouraging others to be more self-assured.

- If you have an important meeting at work, for example, you might approach one of your colleagues afterward and say, "I really admire how good you are at public speaking!" You made the information very clear to comprehend. Thank you a lot!"

- If you have children, you should model this behavior by complimenting them on their attributes rather than their appearance. Instead of saying things like "You look so handsome!" or "You're so beautiful!" you should say things like "You're so intelligent!" or "You're so kind to your friends!"

6. Set a goal for yourself to learn a new skill or complete a difficult task. Trying something different will improve your confidence, and you may be shocked at what you can accomplish. Enroll in a community college class or do something around the house that you've never done before.

- For example, if your car is due for an oil change, you can set a goal for yourself to complete it on your own. Look up videos online and read your owner's manual before doing an oil change with the knowledge you've gained. If you've always wanted to learn a foreign language, enroll in a weekly introductory class and practice at home. You might be surprised by how much you can learn in a matter of months!

7. Participate in activities that you enjoy. Doing stuff that you're good at is one of the easiest ways to feel good about yourself. Sign up for a competitive sport or join a local

enthusiast group to show off your abilities. This will allow you to meet people who share your interests and show that you are more than your appearance.

- If you enjoy bowling, for example, you can join a local bowling league to meet new people and improve your game.

If you like reading, find a book club that meets in your area or close to you and read the book for the next meeting.

Chapter 11: STOP SUGAR CRAVINGS

Every year, the average American woman consumes 48 pounds of added sugar. That works out to four pounds every month! And dental cavities aren't the only potential health problem to be concerned about. Consuming too much sugar increases the chances of developing life-threatening obesity, diabetes, and cardiovascular disease. In reality, a study published in JAMA Internal Medicine showed that people who consumed more added sugar than the recommended daily limit (10 percent of total caloric intake) had a 30 percent higher risk of dying from heart disease.

Ending sugar cravings and reducing added sugar consumption is difficult because sweet foods tempt us at every turn. For many people, eating such foods is a long-standing habit synonymous with comfort or celebration — sugar whispers at you from the grocery store aisles and calls on you from the fridge. The good news is that you can substantially reduce your sugar cravings and reclaim your health by implementing smart sugar strategies.

Why do we crave sugar?

Understanding why cravings occur in the first place — and there are many factors at play — is the first step toward regaining control over sugar. According to Marisa Moore, M.B.A., R.D.N., L.D., a culinary and integrative dietitian, "we crave sugar for a number of reasons, from hormones to behaviors to the psychological effect of simply seeing a decadent donut or a drizzle of caramel." "There is an inherent desire for sweet-tasting foods." Sugar cravings are ingrained in our bodies from a young age. "Among scientists, the assumption appears to be that sweet tastes exist as a way to classify sources of digestible carbohydrates and, more importantly, glucose-based energy," Moore adds. The evolutionary drive to nourish your body is intense and difficult to conquer, so don't be too harsh on yourself if you're having trouble cutting back on sugar — and realize that removing sugar from your diet isn't worth it. "Because humans love sweets, it can be difficult to cut them out completely, and doing so can also lead to feelings of deprivation, which can lead to overindulgence when they get it," Moore explains. This fuels a cycle of shame and guilt, so Moore advises giving yourself some grace during this process.

The problem of sugar

The introduction of the Sugar Tax in the UK has left no doubt in our minds that our Chief Medical Officer believes we will all be healthier if we consumed less sugar.

But what's the actual problem?

Unfortunately, there are plenty. Perhaps this is why previous, less draconian attempts to persuade us to reduce our consumption have failed: we don't fully comprehend the 'why' behind the advice.

So, here are 11 main research-backed reasons why sugar is bad for your health:

1. Sugar promotes weight gain

But why?

To begin with, a significant amount of sugar is 'added' to your regular diet. Processed foods account for the majority of sugar in the average diet.

Sugar is used to enhance the flavor of processed foods. Examine the ingredient labels on the foods in your refrigerator and cupboard. Some of them might surprise you:

- Soft drinks
- Biscuits
- Sweets
- Ketchup
- Sauces
- Ready meals
- Savory snacks
- Cakes
- Yogurts

All of these have sugar added to them, which you then eat or drink.

What does this imply? Unnecessary calories are being consumed!

Another problem is that simple sugars do not provide long-term satisfaction. They have a hit-or-miss effect on your system, leaving you hungry again soon after.

A raft of clinical studies indicates that people who consume more added sugars eat more. 2-5 Complex carbs and protein are much more satisfying and keep you happy for more extended periods.

Finally, simple sugars are high on the Glycaemic Index.

The Glycaemic Index is a food's ability to increase your blood glucose levels after you have eaten.

Foods with a high GI are less satisfying than those with a lower GI. According to one study, teenage boys given high GI foods felt hungrier and consumed 53 percent more calories than those given low GI foods.

Foods with a high GI cause a rise in insulin levels and limit fat breakdown.

Such foods, according to research, can increase fat deposition in the body.

Certain forms of sugars, such as fructose (found in fruits), are primarily converted to fat in the liver.

According to studies, drinking only one sugary beverage a day raises the risk of gaining weight by 60%.

It's important to remember, however, that we're not discussing fruit.

Fruit contains a lot of sugar by itself, but the sugar is absorbed more slowly when you consume a whole piece of fruit.

Fruit provides many the nutrients we need, while added sugars and table sugar have little nutritional value aside from the energy (calories) they provide.

Numerous clinical studies relate sugar intake to weight gain, but one systematic review stands out.

Researchers reviewed almost all major studies that have been done to date that show a correlation between sugar intake and body weight in that review. The following were the outcomes:

Sugar Promotes Weight Gain

Study Design	Total Number of Studies	Studies with a Strong Positive Association Between Sugar Consumption and Weight Gain	Studies with No or Negative Association Between Sugar Consumption and Weight Gain
Cross sectional	15	10	5
Cohort	10	7	3
Clinical Trials	5	5	0

This means that 23 of the 30 studies examined found a connection between sugar intake and weight gain.

2. It raises the risk of developing Type 2 Diabetes.
Sugars, such as sucrose and fructose, have repeatedly been shown to increase the risk of Type 2 Diabetes in studies. Researchers looked at the outcomes of 11 separate studies with a total of 310,819 participants in a review. The findings revealed that people who consume more sugar in their diet are 26% more likely to develop type 2 diabetes.
Insulin is responsible for sugar metabolism, except fructose. It's produced by the beta cells in your pancreas. Long-term sugar consumption raises the risk of developing type 2 diabetes for two reasons.
First, the Korean National Institute of Health claims that chronic sugar consumption is harmful to the pancreas' beta cells. It has the potential to destroy these cells and reduce insulin secretion significantly.
The second and more significant reason is that insulin resistance is increasing. Insulin resistance occurs when your cells do not react appropriately to the insulin generated by your body.
The good news is that diabetes caused by too much sugar can be reversed.
In one study, researchers looked at the impact of sugar reduction on insulin levels in obese women. The researchers discovered that cutting their sugar consumption to 10% of their overall calorie intake improved insulin secretion and sensitivity significantly.

3. Link with Alzheimer's
The human brain is one of the most complex structures known. Unlike other parts of the body, the brain relies heavily on glucose, which can get energy from glucose, proteins, and fats.
Alzheimer's is an age-related brain disorder. It is the weakening of your brain's structural and functional ability.

According to researchers, a strong correlation has been discovered between this disease, sugar consumption, and type 2 diabetes.

Insulin resistance, according to researchers, limits the supply of glucose to the brain. Sugar consumption causes inflammation in the brain, which adds insult to injury.

It also hastens the accumulation of irregular proteins in the brain, which is the hallmark of this condition.

4. Sugar has a detrimental impact on the heart and circulatory system.

Triglycerides are chemicals found in your blood that serve a variety of functions. However, when their levels rise, it raises the risk of high blood pressure, stroke, and heart attack.

Researchers are now trying to figure out how sugar consumption leads to a rise in these chemicals' levels.

Scientists made an incredible observation in a single study.

They looked at how a high sugar, low-fat diet, and low sugar, high fat diet affected the blood's triglyceride levels.

Surprisingly, the low sugar, high-fat diet did not result in a rise in triglyceride levels.

However, with the high-sugar, low-fat diet, they recorded a significant increase in triglycerides' blood levels.

In further research, scientists changed the sugar content of the participants' diets and studied its impact on serum triglyceride levels.

They discovered that those who consumed more sugar had a 46 percent rise in serum triglyceride levels than those who consumed less sugar, who only had a 21 percent increase.

Increased levels of these chemicals in the blood indicate a higher risk of conditions like high blood pressure.

A large body of clinical evidence suggests that eating too much sugar can lead to hypertension.

Researchers discovered in one study that drinking more than one sugary beverage a day increases the risk of developing high blood pressure in the long run.

There is a lack of clinical evidence relating sugar intake to more serious consequences such as heart attack and stroke. However, some research has linked high GI foods to a higher risk of heart attack and stroke.

5. Sugar can throw your hormones off balance

Sugar messes with your hormones.

Affected Hormones	Effect on the Body
Thyroid Hormone	Hypothyroidism: Decrease in thyroid levels, which may lead to weight gain, sluggish mental function, constipation, lethargy, and intolerance to cold. Hyperthyroidism: Increase in thyroid levels, which may lead to weight loss, diarrhea, confusion, body aches, and intolerance to heat.
Growth Hormone	Persistent increases in blood sugar levels and long-term sugar consumption can decrease growth hormone levels and impair children's growth.
Testosterone	Only one-time, sugar intake can decrease testosterone levels by 25 percent. It can lead to erectile poor libido, dysfunction, and infertility.
Oestrogen	Excess sugar can cause estrogen imbalance in females, leading to Polycystic Ovarian Syndrome (PCOS). PCOS leads to infertility and menstrual abnormalities.

6. Sugar can increase toxicity levels in your liver

Sugars, especially fructose, go hard on your liver.

Fructose is primarily metabolised in your liver. When you eat it, it travels to your liver. Instead of being used as energy, it is converted to fat in your liver.

Fructose, according to studies, increases fat deposits in the body, especially in the liver and muscles. Non-alcoholic fatty liver disease is characterized by the accumulation of fat in the liver.

Non-alcoholic fatty liver disease is the first stage of liver failure. If it persists, you can develop full-blown liver failure, which can be fatal.

7. Sugar Rots Your Teeth

Can you recall your mother or grandmother stopping you from eating sweets?

You may have hated it at the time, but it was necessary for your good.

The sugar you eat feeds a lot of bacteria in your mouth. They convert sugar to acid, which eats away at the enamel in your teeth, causing dental problems.

8. Cancer Risk

But that isn't the case. Sugar does more damage to your body than just giving you dental issues.

Newer research indicates that consuming too much sugar increases the risk of various cancers, including pancreatic and small intestine cancer.

This effect is attributed to sugar's ability to tamper with insulin levels, according to scientists.

9. Sugar Hides in Drinks

The satiety properties of a food are based on its form, i.e., whether it is liquid or solid.

Over the past few decades, our eating habits have changed dramatically, but the introduction of sugary beverages and soft drinks is the most significant change.

Researchers conclude that consuming sugary drinks increases the chances of gaining weight more than eating similar solid foods. This is mostly because drinks do not satisfy you for long periods.

In one study, fifteen adult subjects were given 450 calories in sugary beverages or solid foods. The results were evaluated after four weeks.

Researchers discovered that the group consuming fluids had a 17 percent rise in daily calorie consumption and a substantial increase in weight compared to the solid food group.

Whether it is in liquid or solid form - it can lead to weight gain. However, consuming sugary drinks is more likely to cause weight gain than eating solid foods with equal sugar content.

10. It's a Growing Addiction

According to experts, sugar intake has increased 22-fold in the U.S population over the last century.

It's difficult to estimate how much sugar the average American person consumes because sugar is present in almost every edible item.

According to some figures, the average US resident consumes up to 90 grams (or 22 teaspoons) of sugar per day.

There is some disagreement among health authorities on what constitutes a healthy daily sugar intake. However, according to the World Health Organization's (WHO) most recent guidelines, daily added sugar consumption does not exceed 10 percent of total daily calorie intake (or 12 teaspoons).

According to the WHO, cutting sugar consumption to 5 percent of daily calories (or 6 teaspoons) has additional health benefits.

The bottom line is that you should consume no more than 12 teaspoons of added sugar per day (or less).

Sugar is Addictive

11. We're Programmed to Like It

Sugar cravings are real. Simply reading the word "sugar" can cause your mouth to water and flood your brain with neurotransmitters.

Sugar cravings, according to research, share the same brain area as sex - the strongest of all desires.

The question is, do you develop a sweet tooth, or are you born with it.

While your likes and dislikes greatly influence what you eat, you develop a taste for sugar even before you are born.

Scientists now believe that having a "sweet tooth" was crucial to human evolution.

Our ancestors knew that whatever tasted sweet must be good for them. This was the beginning of our sugar addiction.

WAYS TO FIGHT SUGAR CRAVINGS

Do you have an uncontrollable sweet tooth? Here's how to keep the sugar cravings at bay.

Do you find yourself wanting another treat two hours after eating the morning Danish? Do you reach for a candy bar to get through your afternoon slump and then a cola to get through your post-slump slump?

If you've discovered that eating sugary snacks makes you crave more sugary snacks, you are not alone. Eating many simple carbohydrates without any protein or fat as a backup will easily relieve hunger and provide a short-term energy boost, but it can also leave you hungry and wanting more.

How would you put an end to your sugar cravings for good? Here's some professional advice.

Why Do We Crave Sugar?

There are a variety of reasons why we go for sweet treats. That appetite may be hardwired. "Sweet is the first taste humans prefer from birth," says Christine Gerbstadt, RD, MD, a dietitian, and American Dietetic Association spokeswoman and a dietitian. Carbohydrates promote the release of serotonin, a feel-good chemical in the brain. Carbohydrates can be found in a variety of forms, including whole grains, fruits, and vegetables.

According to Susan Moores, MS, RD, a nutrition counselor in St. Paul, Minn., and a registered dietitian, the taste of sugar activates endorphins, which calm and relax us and provide a natural "high."

Sweets taste good, too. And rewarding ourselves with sweet treats strengthens that preference, making you crave it even more. With all that going for it, why wouldn't we crave sugar? The problem occurs when we overindulge in sweet treats, which is simple to do when sugar is added to many processed foods, such as bread, milk, juices, and sauces. The American Heart Association suggests restricting added sugars to about 6 teaspoons per day for women and 9 teaspoons per day.

According to the American Heart Association, Americans eat about 22 teaspoons of added sugars per day on average.

How to Stop Sugar Cravings: 8 Tips to Use Right Now

If you are craving sugar, there are a few things you can do to curb your craving.

• Give in a little. Kerry Neville, MS, RD, a registered dietitian, and ADA spokesperson, recommends eating a tiny fraction of what you're cravings, such as a small cookie or a fun-size candy bar. Allowing yourself to indulge in a small amount of what you enjoy will help you avoid feeling denied. Stick to a 150-calorie limit, according to Neville.

• Combine foods. You can still fill yourself up and fulfill a sugar addiction if stopping at a cookie or a baby candy bar seems unlikely. "I enjoy combining a craving food with a healthy one," says Neville. "For example, I love chocolate, so I'll dip a banana in chocolate sauce to satisfy my cravings, or I'll mix some almonds with chocolate chips." You'll also satisfy a craving and get nutritious nutrients from those good-for-you foods as a bonus.

• Go cold turkey. For certain people, eliminating all simple sugars works, but "the first 48 to 72 hours are difficult," according to Gerbstadt. Some people report that going cold turkey reduces their cravings after a few days; others report that they still crave sugar and train their taste buds to be satisfied with less over time.

• Grab some gum. If you want to stop giving in to a sugar craving, registered dietitian Dave Grotto, RD, LDN, recommends chewing a stick of gum. "Chewing gum has been shown in studies to relieve food cravings," Grotto says.

• Reach for fruit. Keep fruit handy for when sugar cravings hit. You will get nutrients and fiber along with some sweetness. Judy Chambers, LCSW, CAS, a licensed addiction expert, recommends stocking up on foods like nuts, seeds, and dried fruits. "Keep them close at hand so you can reach for them instead of the old [sugary] something."

• Get up and go. When you have a sugar craving, walk away. "Take a stroll around the block or do something to change the scenery," to divert your attention away from the food you're craving, Neville suggests.

• Choose quality over quantity. "If you need a sugar splurge, pick a delicious, decadent sugary food," Moores advises. But keep it small. Instead of a king-sized candy bar, Moores suggests choosing a beautiful dark chocolate truffle and "savoring every taste — slowly." Grotto agrees. "Don't swear off favorites; you'll just come back for more. Learn to integrate small quantities into your diet when focusing on filling your stomach with [healthier] less sugary choices."

• Eat regularly. According to Moores, waiting too long between meals can cause you to choose sugary, fatty foods to satisfy your hunger. Instead, Grotto recommends eating every three to five hours to keep blood sugar steady and prevent "irrational eating behavior." What are your best bets? Moores recommends eating protein- and fiber-rich foods like whole grains and produce.

However, won't eating more often lead to overeating? Not if you follow Neville's advice to break up your meals. For example, save some yogurt for a mid-morning snack and eat part of your breakfast — maybe a slice of toast with peanut butter. "Break up lunch the same way to help prevent a mid-afternoon slump," Neville advises.

How to Stop Sugar Cravings: 5 Tips for the Long Term

One of the most effective ways to manage sugar cravings is to stop them before they start. To help you do that:

• Avoid artificial sweeteners at all costs. Artificial sweeteners might seem like a good idea. Still, according to Grotto, author of 101 Foods That Could Save Your Life, "they don't lessen sugar cravings and haven't shown a positive impact on our obesity epidemic."

• Reward yourself for overcoming your sugar cravings. Your reward may be substantial or small. Remember why you're working on it, and then reward yourself on each move you complete.

• Slow down. Chambers recommends focusing on your sugar cravings and thinking about what you're consuming for a week. Diet mayhem often results from a lack of planning. Slow down, plan, and "eat what you want to eat, rather than eating when you are desperate," Chambers suggests.

• Get support. Many people turn to sweet foods when they are depressed, angry, or stressed. However, food does not fix emotional problems. Consider whether emotions cause your sugar cravings, and whether you need help in getting alternative solutions to those emotional issues.

• Mix it up. You may need more than one strategy to combat sugar cravings. One week you may find success with one tactic, but another week can necessitate a different approach. What's essential, according to Gerbstadt, is to "have a 'bag of tricks' to try." To control sugar cravings, Neville recommends "figuring out what works for you."

Finally, go easy on yourself. It may take some time to overcome your sugar cravings. "It is difficult to shift any system — whether it is the world economy or your eating," Chambers says.

FOODS THAT CAN FIGHT SUGAR CRAVINGS

Sugar cravings are very common, especially in women.
In reality, up to 97 percent of women and 68 percent of men say they've had a food craving, including sugar cravings.
Sugar cravings trigger a powerful desire to consume something sweet and make it difficult to maintain self-control around food.
This can lead to binge eating or calorie overconsumption, sometimes regularly.
Fortunately, there are certain things you can do to alleviate the discomfort.
Here are foods that will help you overcome your sugar cravings.

1. Fruit

When most people are hungry for sweets, they turn to high-fat, high-sugar foods like chocolate.

Swapping junk food for fruit when you're craving something sweet can provide the sweet hit you're looking for while also putting a stop to your craving.

Fruit is naturally sweet, but it also contains a lot of nutritious plant compounds and fiber, so you can get your fix while staying healthy.

Eat fruits with higher sugar content, such as mangoes or grapes, to ensure it hits the spot.

If you're hungry, mix some yogurt in with your fruit to make a more satisfying snack.

2. Berries

Berries are a delicious and nutritious way to curb sugar cravings.

They have a sweet flavor, but their high fiber content implies they are low in sugar.

If you believe your sugar cravings are due to habit rather than hunger, this could make them a great choice. For instance, you might crave sweet foods while you are watching TV.

Berries are also high in plant compounds, which have powerful antioxidant and anti-inflammatory effects.

This means they can reduce risk factors for chronic diseases such as heart disease and diabetes.

However, they are rich in fiber and sugar-free. Eating berries regularly can also help.

Assist in the prevention of heart disease and diabetes.

3. Dark Chocolate

Chocolate is one of the most common foods people eat when people have a sugar craving. This is particularly true for women.

However, if you have a chocolate craving, you can make a healthier option by opting for dark chocolate.

Dark chocolate is chocolate that contains more than 70 percent cocoa. It also contains healthy plant substances known as polyphenols.

The antioxidant and anti-inflammatory properties of these polyphenols have been shown in several studies to help enhance heart health markers.

Dark chocolate, like normal chocolate, contains sugar and fat, but you can only eat a couple of squares to satisfy your craving.

4. Snack Bars

Snack bars aren't all nutritious, and some are particularly high in fat and sugar.

If you are craving a sweet treat, there are some nice, healthier options available.

Instead of table sugar, search for a snack bar made with whole oats and sweetened with fresh or dried fruit.

Keep an eye out for bars that are high in so-called "healthy" sugars like honey, agave syrup, or coconut sugar. These are still added sugar, which is harmful to your health.

Whole foods have been used to make the best bars. Even if they are still very sweet, they are likely to be higher in fiber and provide more beneficial nutrients.

Alternatively, you might use a recipe like this to make your balanced snack bar.

5. Chia Seeds

Chia seeds contain various nutrients, including omega-3 fatty acids, soluble dietary fiber, and several healthy plant compounds.

Soluble fiber accounts for around 40 percent of chia seeds. This type of fiber absorbs water quickly and expands in your gut to form a jelly-like substance, making you feel fuller for longer and prevent sugar cravings.

Chia seeds are also flexible, so if you're looking for a sweet treat, consider making a chia pudding like this one.

6. Sugar-Free Chewing Gum or Mints

Gum chewing will help you curb your sugar cravings. Artificially sweetened gum or mints have a sweet taste but have few calories and no sugar.

Although the evidence is mixed, some studies have shown that chewing gum can help regulate hunger, cravings, and carbohydrate intake later in the day.

Chewing gum after meals is healthy for your teeth as well as helping you battle the sugar craving.

7. Legumes

Legumes like beans, chickpeas, and lentils are great plant-based sources of fiber and protein.

One cup of lentils (198 grams) contains about 18 grams of protein and 16 grams of fiber.

Both of these nutrients are thought to help you feel more satisfied. Thus, including legumes in your diet can help you feel fuller and reduce sugar cravings caused by hunger.

In line with this, a recent study discovered that eating lentils can help you lose weight.

This may be due to the short-term beneficial effects that legumes have on appetite.

8. Yogurt

Yogurt is a low-fat, high-protein snack that is also high in calcium.

Yogurt can also be a healthy snack to help balance your appetite and control your cravings.

According to one study, healthy-weight women who had high-protein Greek yogurt for an afternoon snack were less hungry and consumed less later in the day than those who had a lower-protein snack or no snack at all.

The healthiest choice for yogurt is one that is free of added sugar and contains live cultures.

9. Dates

Dates are the dried fruit of the date palm tree. They are very sweet and highly nutritious.

Even though they have been dried, they are a great source of potassium, iron, fiber, and beneficial plant compounds.

If you eat a few dates instead of a soda or candy, you'll get a sweet fix while still getting some good nutrients.

For a sweet and crunchy treat, consider mixing them with nuts such as almonds.

Keep in mind that dates are very sweet, so limit yourself to one portion at a time or three dates.

10. Sweet Potatoes

Sweet potatoes are nutrient-dense, sweet, and very filling. They're mainly carbs, but they're also high in fiber and various vitamins and minerals like vitamin A, vitamin C, and potassium.

Some people get sugar cravings because they are not eating enough throughout the day.

Including a carb source like sweet potatoes in your meals will help you fight this by adding calories and making your meals more balanced while providing you the sweet taste you are craving.

Try roasting them with cinnamon and paprika, as in this recipe, for a delicious treat.

Having the odd sweet treat is fine for most people, so you should not feel guilty if you indulge occasionally.

If you find yourself craving sugar daily or feeling out of control around sweet foods, it's time to reconsider your diet.

If you need something sweet, consider replacing some of your sugary treats with some of the healthier choices on this list.

Chapter 12: HOW TO BE SUCCESSFUL WITH ANY DIET PLAN

While I recommend macro counting and flexible dieting as effective methods for losing weight and achieving fitness goals, there are several other to diet and be successful at it. Some people eat Paleo, and others eat low-carb, and even others eat whatever they want as long as they keep track of their calories. Any diet that helps you to eat in a calorie deficit can help you lose weight.

Yes, some diet methods are better than others in terms of restriction and ensuring that the body gets the nutrients it requires, but it's not the approach that prevents success; rather, it's the internal dialogue that brings most diets to a halt.

When dieting, the most important thing to pay attention to is what's going on in your head.

Three Essential Skills For Diet Success

1. Believe that you can change.

Let me explain before you write me off as some new age wooshu guy.

People who have changed their bodies had a deep confidence in their ability to improve. They knew exactly what they wanted and how to get it, so they went for it.

I've discovered that to excel in every undertaking, one must believe in oneself. Of course, there are moments when we stumble into amazing things, but I've noticed that this is rare.

I've seen a lot of people who have tried and struggled to lose weight for years. This makes them feel like they've failed miserably, and they're unable to believe that this time will be any different. One of my first tasks is to help them trust in themselves and the process. They must invest in the journey, not just give it a "try."

How much of our potential will we unlock if we only give dieting a shot rather than believing that anything will change? If you think you can do a thing or think you can not do a thing, you are right. – Henry Ford.

For me, this is something I've had to focus on in several areas of my life, including my fitness journey.

I was never an athlete in high school, and my grandfather once told me that I had fat thighs like my mother. It wasn't until I was in my 30s that I began to believe I could change my body from average to muscular.

If you want to succeed at dieting, you must first believe that you can succeed.

2. Look for inspiration and encouragement

We usually don't just stumble into a greater sense of belief; we have to fight for it.

There is one thing that has helped me grow confidence more than anything else...

Testimonials.

I had seen so many before and after transformations that I convinced myself that if they could do it, so could I. We must train ourselves to believe that everything is possible.

As I previously said, there are several methods for changing your body – just make sure that whatever approach you choose is backed by real-life stories of people just like you and me who have achieved success.

It's also the only thing that can get us through a hard patch when we doubt whether or not this thing works at all. I know because I've done it several times before.

Along with this, it's important to surround yourself with people who can inspire you to keep going rather than knock you down.
Find people who can cheer you on and help pick you up when you get tired, whether they be friends, family, a trainer, a coach, or even members of your class.
Encouragement is powerful!

3. Tell Yourself the Right Stories
When we want to change our bodies, we can make up the most bizarre stories, right?
These stories have an impact on what we believe, how we act, and who we become. Some people refuse to lose weight because they feel they won't be able to. And, when they can't lose weight, they make up a lie to explain themselves.
Overcoming the stories we tell ourselves is one of the most difficult aspects of making some progress in life.

- "It's impossible for me to eat better."
- "I'm big-boned."
- "I've always been fat; I can never change."
- "I have the fat gene."
- "I don't have enough time."

These thoughts are often referred to as limiting beliefs.
Whatever you call them, one thing is certain: GET RID OF THEM!
You don't always need to change your strategy; sometimes, all you need to do is change your story.
Here are three questions to ask yourself to help you develop a better story.
1. What stories are holding you back?
We also have our narratives. Some of them are beneficial and help us succeed. Others are harmful and impede our progress.

What stories or beliefs do you need to let go of to move forward?
This move requires you to be honest with yourself. It's about confronting the excuses and calling them out for what they are. Answering this question can be daunting because it requires you to face outright lies that you tell yourself.
For example. "I haven't done it because I don't have enough… Time. Money. Energy."
Whatever they are, jot them down on a piece of paper and make a list.

2. What stories will move you forward?
Now that we've looked at what's been holding you back, we need to substitute those beliefs with positive ones.
What helpful stories will you start telling yourself?
e.g.
- "I possess more than enough energy.'
- "I have all the time I need."
- "I can do this."

I'm not talking about positive affirmations, though they can be helpful, simply controlling the thoughts, you think daily.
What if you replaced every negative story you told yourself with a positive one that helped you move forward?

3. How can you recall these better stories?
I have a list of things taped to the bathroom mirror that I read while I brush my teeth. They serve as a constant reminder of who I am and what I am capable of. It's a little cheesy, but it's crazy effective.
- Maybe you will have them in a note on your phone.
- Maybe you have a supercomputer for a brain and can simply remember everything.
- Maybe you will keep a card in your wallet.

Whatever it is, whether tangible or not, make it a focus.

Working on nurturing the basic belief that change is possible will transform your life!

Chapter 13: SPEED UP YOUR METABOLISM

Our metabolisms are held responsible for a lot of things. "Metabolism" is a buzzword we throw around with our girlfriends when we're irritated. Our inability to mainline chocolate without putting on weight? Metabolism. Our general fatigue? Metabolism. Those seven pounds that just won't budge? Metabolism. But do you know what your metabolism is and what it even does?

"Metabolism" is described as "all the chemical processes that occur continuously within the body to keep you alive and your organs working normally, such as breathing, digesting food, repairing cells, and" according to the NHS website. Our bodies need the energy to perform all of these metabolic processes, and our basal metabolic rate (BMR) is the number of calories our bodies need to keep us alive. "A slow metabolism is more accurately defined as a low BMR." While we should probably change our attention from wanting to speed up our metabolism to wanting to increase our BMR if we want to be accurate, at the end of the day, we all just want to know how to lose more extra weight, right? Here's how to do it.

Eat a Metabolism-Boosting Breakfast

There's some controversy about whether eating breakfast like a king, lunch like a prince, and dinner like a pauper is the key to losing weight.

I can happily eat breakfast, lunch, and dinner like a king and not be bloated (which is a shame). Rather than thinking about your weight, the type of foods you put on your breakfast plate significantly impacts your metabolism. According to a study, you should include low-GL (low-sugar) and high-protein foods in your breakfast if you want to fire up your system. Consider savory flavors and lean proteins such as chicken (yes, for breakfast) or eggs.

When it comes to basic cardio (not including HIIT), you just burn calories when you're active, but HIIT and strength training increase your metabolism for hours afterward, increasing fat burn for much longer than the time you were working. However, you may well like a jaunt on a treadmill over a heavy HIIT session. One study showed that an intermittent incline (moving up and down on the treadmill as if running over hills) will help to improve your metabolism.

Drink Green Tea

"Coffee bean are a difficult seed to crack. Your morning coffee is rich in antioxidants, but it's also related to cortisol overproduction and adrenal exhaustion," says Kelly LeVeque, founder of Be Well by Kelly and health coach. "Drinking brewed green tea, on the other hand, is a good way to get caffeine while also giving your body EGCG (epigallocatechin gallate), a metabolism-boosting ingredient. Consider the beWELL method: Start your day with a cup of coffee, then switch to green tea in the afternoon.

Avoid all sodas, and calorie-laden coffee drinks since high cortisol levels induced by excessive caffeine are more likely to trigger weight gain around your waist."

Factor in Fiber

Increasing your fiber intake to 30 grams a day can be just as good as counting calories for weight loss. What do you mean by that? Since fiber is indigestible, according to Tanya Zuckerbrot, MS, RD, founder of the F-Factor Diet, consuming a diet rich in high-fiber foods improves metabolism. Soluble fiber absorbs water as it is digested and keeps you fuller for longer, while insoluble fiber simply passes through the system, assisting us in passing our food.

"The body can't absorb fiber, but it tries," she tells Fox News Lifestyle. "The body expends more calories trying to absorb and remove fiber than it does for most foods. As a result, digesting high-fiber foods burns more calories than digesting processed carbohydrates."

Most fiber contains both insoluble and soluble fibers. Foods higher in insoluble fiber include beans, cauliflower, wheat bran, and apples. While soluble fiber is found in oat bran, artichokes, and brown rice, among other foods.

Get Your Micronutrients

While a healthy metabolism equals a healthy body, metabolic syndrome may result in diabetes, weight gain, and heart disease. Of course, exercise and a balanced diet will help avoid this, but if you're in a rush and your exercises and healthy meals have fallen by the wayside, make sure you're supplementing with the right micronutrients. Certain vitamins and minerals have been discovered to aid in the maintenance of a balanced metabolism. Although we can get these from a varied diet, it's also worth supplementing with a supplement. Vitamins E and C, according to one study, are important for a healthy metabolism. Vitamin D is also important in preventing metabolic syndrome, and since we live in a country where the sun doesn't always shine, it's important to take it every day, regardless of your diet.

Build Muscle

Strength training, as previously said, is the secret to burning more fat at rest (in other words, for raising your BMR). Lean muscle can help you increase your BMR by speeding up your metabolism. While cardio, especially HIIT, will help you lose weight, "HIIT training has been shown to increase metabolism for up to eight hours after training," says LeVeque. Strength training will help you gain lean muscle. She claims that "weight-lifting has been shown to improve the burn for up to 39 hours."

"In general, men have a faster metabolism because they have more muscle mass... and less body fat than women, which is why their daily calorie allowance is higher," according to the NHS website. So, what does all of this mean? I time to start taking training tips from the boys.

Chapter 14: THINK THIN

WAYS OF THINKING THIN
When the first buds of spring pop out, motivation to lose weight often hits an all-time high, signaling that bathing suit season is not far behind. And while the need for exercise and healthier eating isn't getting around, long-term weight loss starts in your head. Experts say that having the correct attitude can help you think that you are thin.
Says Pamela Peeke, MD, author of Fit to Live, if you want to succeed in weight loss, you need to "cut the mental fat, and that will lead to cutting the waistline fat," "Look at the patterns and habits in your life that you are dragging around with you that get in the way of success."
Everyone has excuses of their own. Most people do fine until something happens when they try to improve their lifestyle and diet — whether it's work pressure, family problems, or something else. Whatever your problem is, if you want to be successful, the trend needs to change.
I want to encourage people to recognize these trends, fix the real problems so that they can move forward and be able to better their well-being, "I want to empower people to identify these patterns, deal with the real issues, so they can move on and be able to succeed at improving their health,"
Dieting does not mean that you are unable to snack. For smart snacking ideas, take this quiz.
To Think Yourself Thin, Have Patience
Wanting too much, too soon, is one big mental barrier to weight loss. With its instant messages, PDAs, and digital cameras, Blame blames it on our instant-gratification society: Weight loss is too sluggish to please most dieters.

Losers want immediate results. ... While it took them years to gain weight, they have little patience with the prescribed 1-2 pounds per week once they decide to lose weight, "Losers want immediate results. ... Even though it took them years to gain weight, once they decide to lose weight, they have no patience with the recommended 1-2 pounds per week,"

But you will get the best results as you slowly lose weight. Sass reminds her clients that they often lose water or lean tissue, not fat when they lose weight too fast.

"When you lose lean tissue, metabolism slows down, making it even harder to lose weight," she says.

Think Thin: 8 Strategies

With these eight strategies, get that overweight mentality out of your head and start thinking like a thin person:

1. Thin Image of Yourself.

Picture yourself thin if you want to be thin. Visualize your future self, down the road for six months to a year, and think about how good without the extra pounds you'll look and feel. As a reminder of what you are working towards, dig up old photographs of your thinner self and place them in a place. Ask yourself what you were doing back then that today you could incorporate into your lifestyle. Peeke advises, think about activities you would like to do, but you cannot because of your weight.

"To break old habits, you need to see yourself in a positive light," Peeke says.

2. Have realistic hopes.

The number is often realistically attainable when doctors ask their patients how much they want to weigh. Peeke has her patients identify a realistic weight range, not a single number. "I ask them to look ahead 12 months, and would they be happier being 12 or 24 pounds thinner?" she says, "It only amounts to 1-2 pounds per month, which is doable, sustainable, and manageable in the context of career and family." She suggests after six months, reevaluating your weight goal.

3. Make Small Goals.

Create a list of smaller targets to help you meet your goals for weight loss. These mini-goals should be things that can boost your lifestyle without creating chaos in your life, such as:

- Eating more fruit and vegetables regularly.
- Having at least 30 minutes a day with some form of physical activity.
- Drinking alcohol on weekends only.
- Eating low-fat popcorn rather than candy,
- Ordering a side salad rather than french fries.
- Being able to walk up a stair flight without gasping for respiration.

"We all know that change is hard, and it is especially difficult if you try to make too many changes, so start small and gradually make lifestyle improvements," Sass suggests.
4. Get Support.
We all need help, especially during difficult times. Find a friend, family member, or support group that you can regularly interact with. Studies show that people associated with others do better than dieters who want to go it alone, whether in person or online.
5. Create a Detailed Action Plan.
Sass recommends that every night, for the next day, you prepare your nutritious meals and exercise. Planning is 80% of the war. Results can follow if you're prepared with a comprehensive plan.
Plan your fitness as if you were going to make an appointment, "Schedule your fitness like you would an appointment," "Pack up dried fruits, veggies, or meal replacement bars so you won't be tempted to eat the wrong kinds of foods."
Building such steps into your life makes your health a priority, and gradually these healthy habits will become a normal part of your life.
6. Yourself the Reward.

Pat yourself on the back with a film tour, a manicure, or something else that will make you feel good about your achievements (other than food rewards).

"Reward yourself after you have met one of your mini-goals or lost 5 pounds or a few inches around your waist, so you recognize your hard work and celebrate the steps you are taking to be healthier," says Peeke.

7. Ditch Old Habits.

Old habits die hard, but if you want to be good at weight loss, you can't continue to do it the way you used to.

"Slowly but surely, try to identify where you are engaging in behaviors that lead to weight gain and turn them around with little steps that you can easily handle without feeling deprived," says Sass.

For example, start by changing your snack from a bag of cookies or chips to a fruit piece if you are an evening couch potato. Try consuming just a calorie-free soda the next night. Finally, when you watch television, you will begin doing exercises.

Another way to start ditching your bad habits: get rid of your kitchen's enticing, empty-calorie foods and substitute them with healthy choices.

8. Just keep track.

Weigh regularly and maintain journals that describe what you eat, how much you work out, your thoughts, and your measurements and weight. Studies show that it helps encourage good habits and reduce unhealthy ones by keeping track of this knowledge. It could help you stop the piece of cake by simply recognizing that you monitor your food intake!

"Journals are a form of accountability … that help reveal which strategies are working," Peeke says. "When you are accountable, you are less likely to have food disassociations or be 'asleep at the meal.'"

Chapter 15: THE SURPRISING LINK BETWEEN PLEASURE AND WEIGHT LOSS

1. Can Your Way Smile Slim?

It seems like a straightforward formula: diet plus exercise equals success in weight loss. But the mental side, which is just as important, is what is often ignored. In your life, how you manage stress and depression can make or break your bikini-body goals. There are real chemical processes taking place that influence the way your body responds to temptations, from the donuts on the conference table to the desire to sleep instead of hitting the gym, whether you're nervous about work or coping with a devastating breakup. Any type of depression, no matter how mild, affects mood, thought, appetite, and behavior-controlled neurotransmitters, making you more likely to eat poorly, miss exercise, and gain weight. [Tweet the truth! Likewise, high levels of stress cause the body to release the hormone cortisol, making us want energy and warmth (often in the form of pizza and cupcakes). This leads to a high level of dopamine induced by sugar, then the inevitable crash that causes you to look for even more dopamine, and so on. Then all those extra empty calories are accumulated in your body, most often in the form of belly fat.

Of course, it's far easier said than done to cope with life's frustrating and saddening circumstances. After all, by buying your salmon or taking a bubble bath, you can't fix all your issues. However, these ten tips will help you combat anxiety, increase serotonin, and release endorphins, all of which will produce a happier mood, a healthier mind, and a slimmer body.

And for even more slim-down secrets, in our latest book, The Bikini Body Diet, check out Shape's exclusive strategy for a beach-ready body.

2. Flash a Smile

According to a new report in Psychological Science, the simple act of smiling is an immediate stress-buster. You can even do it at any time, assuming that at the moment, the boss is not chewing you out.

3. Drink Up

According to a Journal of Nutrition study, if you're dehydrated, you're more likely to feel more tired and depressed and have less energy, so staying hydrated with water is important (plus: no calories!). Water may not wash away your issues, but it is an important part of coping with life's tasks and achieving your physical and emotional goals to maintain energy levels.

4. Seek Peace

Find an activity that will allow you to do mini-meditations, including outdoor hiking or walking. Research published in BMC Public Health found that it was more vital for a 20-minute walk outdoors twice a week than doing the same workout indoors. But it can help you slow down even by doing things like preparing a nutritious meal. Take the time to slice, smell the scents, and participate in the cooking process, and it can serve as a mind-cleanser. [Have this tip tweeted!]

5. Stretch It Out

With a deep forward bend, get your entire body in on the fun. This step is ideal because it decompresses the spine and increases circulation, which allows the upper body and your mind to relieve tension. Stand with your feet hip-width apart to do one, then slightly bend your knees and fold your body forward. Grip the opposite elbows and lower your head; keep it for a minute.

Another good way to relieve tension is to contract your muscles and then release them because, after being under tension, they are more able to relax completely: take a few deep breaths and then contract your right arm as tightly as you can, holding it for two or three seconds. Relax fully as you exhale and let your arm drop. You can replicate it with other parts of the body and even the whole body.

6. Power Down

A British study found that reviewing e-mails and messages compulsively would cause anxiety. Take 15-minute breaks from your phone every hour, and check out these eight quick steps to do a digital detox without feeling like you're missing out if you want to try to unplug even further.

7. Choc It Up

The building blocks of eating for a beach-ready body have already been covered, but a few of our favorite bikini-friendly foods have been specifically shown to improve mood. [Tweet the list here! To keep those happy chemicals high and the hungry ones low, include more of these on your plate:

Walnuts can boost serotonin levels, which helps to put you in a good mood.

Approximately 40 grams of dark chocolate made of 75 percent cocoa lowers stress hormone levels.

Chickpeas contain folate, a B vitamin necessary for dopamine production, a neurotransmitter most associated with pleasure.

Avocados contain B vitamins, which help create serotonin that feels good. They have potassium as well, which can help lower blood pressure.

Seeds of sunflower have loads of magnesium. Your dopamine levels can be reduced by a lack of this nutrient, making you feel more stressed and anxious.

8. Seafood

Omega-3 fats are present in fatty, coldwater fish such as salmon, tuna, and sardines, making you feel calmer. In one study, individuals who ate foods high in omega-3s regularly were 20 percent less anxious than those who did not. According to a study by Ohio State University, people who took an omega-3 supplement for 12 weeks saw their anxiety levels drop 20 percent.

9. Move It!

Countless studies have shown how some serious mental health benefits are provided by exercise. In our Bikini Body Workout, making the moves will not only help you trim your trouble zones but will also help increase feel-good endorphins and energy, which will greatly enhance your mindset.

10. Buddy Up

Encourage a friend or member of the family to join you on your bikini body quest. Having a system of social support improves levels of oxytocin, the feel-good hormone. In the form of a hobby, a good conversation, or hanging out with the family, satisfying your dopamine system may come. What this does is change your dopamine system to derive satisfaction, not nacho chips, from other things in your life.

11. Let Others Know

We don't suggest taking out an ad on your journey in the paper or blogging, but there is evidence that sharing your diet and exercise goals is an effective way to stay on track. Tell one, two, five, or ten people who can relate to what you're going through when you feel like downing a pint of Ben and Jerry's or who can act as a sounding board. You will not only keep depression at bay by including others in your journey, but you will also be using the very tool that may very well be the key to successfully following through on a weight loss plan: the responsibility that comes from involving other people.

Chapter 16: HOW TO GO BACK TO NORMAL EATING AFTER WEIGHT LOSS OR A DIET

Losing weight isn't easy. Weight loss also typically requires a stricter diet than you may be used to, in addition to a regular workout plan with Aaptiv.

However, once you're in a groove, habits begin to form, and your plan for weight loss becomes second nature. Then, returning to a regular eating pattern and maintaining the loss becomes the hard part.

When you're in a short-term, rigid eating pattern, the normal daily eating pitfalls are not as much a problem as a problem. Seeing the weight fall off, you're on a roll, and the diet keeps your choices in check.

But it's much more difficult to navigate food choices once you've reached your goal weight and are looking to move to a normal way of eating after weight loss.

By making lifestyle changes that work for you, maintaining your weight loss is the most successful way. It can be hard to transition from dieting to regular eating. But the following tips on eating after weight loss will help you move to a healthy maintenance diet successfully.

Eat mindfully.

Conscious eating habits are incorporated into meals. Make a pact with yourself that you will avoid eating mindlessly. This involves the kind of snacks off the radar that you don't even know how much you eat. Mindful eating enables you to better process your body's signals and stops when your body says it's full. Make mealtime the main event to do this. Set up your table, turn off your television and phone, and enjoy your meal. Take the time to pay tribute to the food and all it takes to bring it to your plate. Think of how it has been cultivated, harvested, and prepared.

Slow your food down and savor each bite. Allow yourself to think about the food's scent, texture, and taste. Set your utensil down between bites as you chew, and after several bites, stop for a drink.

Mindful eating may be a challenge for you, as in our culture, we tend to eat on the run and value quick meals. Be patient and give yourself time to learn how to change eating habits for a lifetime.

Expect setbacks.

Yep, there are moments when you just can't say no to the extra helping of a cake, you just have a little too much to drink, or you lose control of your appetizer table. Life is that. The most important method for sustaining weight loss is learning how to treat dietary slips and get back on track.

If you have a bad food day, when your head hits the pillow, be done with it. The next morning, you can still start new. These three doughnuts are history. It would only derail your self-esteem and motivation by hanging onto any feelings of shame associated with your diet. As a delicious detour, chalk them up and get back on the safe eating train. Besides, those donuts (or whatever your slip food was) probably left you feeling lousy-a strong reinforcement to stay on track now that your regular diet consists of nutritious food.

Avoid rigid eating after weight loss.

The ambulatory dietitian at the Watertown Regional Medical Center in Wisconsin, Kris Bennett, RDN, CD, reminds us to avoid an excessively restrictive diet. "Bennett says, "Restricting or avoiding certain foods are typical pitfalls. She explains that they appear to crave it when someone limits a certain food and can even over-eat other foods trying to stop the one they crave. They can even gorge on the desired food eventually.

Enable throughout the week for small, portion-controlled quantities of favorite foods. You will find that if your budget for the food in your diet and do not make it a daily routine, it will not have the power to derail your healthy eating.

Keep a food journal.

During a diet, the last thing you probably feel like doing is writing down what you are eating. However, keeping a food log may make the difference between success or failure during the first weeks of maintenance. It makes you stop and take the time to pay attention to your diet by writing down everything you consume. And maintaining a log is necessary if the scale begins to creep up, to make adjustments to your caloric intake.

Portion control is your friend.

Over the past decades, the typical serving size has steadily increased for bagels, muffins, and restaurant meals. So how do you decide what a typical serving size is? In comparison with other objects, learn to estimate. For example, one cup is approximately the size of a tennis ball, and the size of a deck of cards should be a serving of meat or fish.

By filling the serving ware with water and measuring it, or using dry foods such as oatmeal or rice to fill and measure, determine your bowls and cups' actual content size. It always takes time to measure it, rather than just pouring, when adding oil to a dish while cooking or dressing.

As a guide to meal portion size, Bennett has her customers use aids such as choosemyPlate.gov. It takes the guesswork out of portions and makes determining how much you should eat after weight loss so much easier.

Eat only when you're hungry.

To learn the difference between actual hunger and eating stress or boredom, pay close attention to your body's signals. Try to determine if your body feels hungry (your stomach is growling) or if your hunger is an emotional response. This may at first be a hard thing to determine. It may take time to learn true indications of hunger versus old eating habits of the stress response. The first step is to become aware of the signs, avoid an immediate reaction (such as grabbing a donut and eating it before considering whether you're really hungry), and make healthier choices.

You'll need to find constructive substitutes for it if food has been a source of emotional support. Working with a psychologist who has experience with mental eating disorders can be very helpful. She can provide resources to substitute emotional eating effectively with healthy choices and provide the required help while you make this transition.

Eat protein at each meal.

Protein can help minimize your appetite by reducing a hormone responsible for hunger, allowing you to feel full faster and remain satisfied longer. Include in every meal at least 20 grams of protein. To help give them staying power, make sure that your snacks also have protein.

Ideally, about 30 percent of your daily diet would consist of protein. Pick low-fat, lean sources (like these), such as fish, lean meat and poultry cuts, and low-fat dairy products. In their diet, most adults do not receive enough protein and need to increase their intake, especially as they age, making it a key part of every meal.

Get your sleep.

Studies have shown that not getting enough sleep can disrupt hunger signals from your body. Your body becomes less glucose-sensitive when you don't get enough quality sleep. While the appetite control hormone leptin is reduced, the hunger hormone ghrelin is increased. In people who do not get adequate levels of sleep, there is an increased risk of obesity. So, if you have a hard time getting eight hours of sleep every night, try to make the changes below.

With the time you go to sleep and get up, stay as consistent as possible. Don't sleep on weekends anymore, thinking it will help you catch up. That'll just disrupt the sleep schedule of your brain.

Shut down all electronic displays several hours before bedtime.

Make the sleeping room-friendly by adding blackout shades if there is a problem with the outside light. Remove any other light sources (electronic alarm clocks, phone chargers).

If you're sensitive to noise, try wearing earplugs. Many kinds of earplugs are available, so try them out to find those that are comfortable.

Turn the room temperature downwards. Research has shown that maintaining the temperature at night between 60-67 degrees increases sleep quality.

If you can not sleep, make it a rule after your evening meal that the kitchen is off-limits. A bad habit can be formed by compensating for not sleeping with food.

It does count calories.

It is a bit of a dance to find your regular calorie maintenance standard. But you'll find your sweet spot with patience and time. Keep in mind that everyone has their unique metabolism and the number of calories necessary for weight maintenance. For example, somebody who is more active should consume more calories than someone less active.

The path to effective weight maintenance is by making positive changes in lifestyle and remaining consistent with those changes. Changing lifelong patterns takes time, so be patient with yourself, and keep your workouts in line with your Aaptiv app. And if you backslide, remember that you can get your next meal back on track.

Chapter 17: MEDITATION AT HOME

Meditation is an efficient technique that for centuries has been around. People who constantly meditate discover that short-term and long-term benefits exist. For example, meditators tend to enjoy a reduction in stress and anxiety, enhanced well-being, and, in certain instances, better sleep and overall health soon after they start sitting. Meditators can better understand how the mind acts and how to deal with their brains in the long term.

Serious meditators, until recently, usually belonged to one of two groups. Either they entered an ashram or monastery and dedicated their lives to practice, or they left behind the hustle-bustle of worldly life and found shelter in the serenity of isolated hermitages. But inside our daily lifestyle, we should find a way of meditating. Nowadays, however, many people who lead active lives can devote time and energy to meditation because they are persuaded of the advantages, such as work, family, education, etc. Some do their regular group meditation sessions, but many more are at home meditating now.

What is the best way to meditate at home?

Choosing a meditation technique that you can look forward to is the first thing to do. While practice involves constancy and discipline, meditation shouldn't feel like work. You'll soon be able to find the perfect balance between too rigid and too comfortable with the right tool.

Next, we have some helpful tips here:

1. Focus on your motivation

Do you meditate because you want to deal with stress, get better sleep, or cope with chronic pain? If so, guided meditation, calming meditation, or chanting will do you good. Looking to gain insights into the mind, are you? This is the real purpose of meditation on mindfulness and perception. Is your main aim to cultivate characteristics such as tolerance, empathy, and generosity? Meditation on appreciation is a healthy choice (if you can do a morning gratitude meditation, it can benefit your whole day). Would you like to go deeper into your engagement with the Divine Presence? There, spiritual practice will carry you.

There are several legitimate meditation forms out there. You'll know which ones are right for you when you know why you're interested in meditating at home.

2. Start small and work up your way

While learning how to meditate at home, starting with small, manageable sessions is important. Three minutes, even, will make a difference. It may sound super short, but for some beginners, sitting in awareness feels like forever for a few minutes. Starting with brief sessions also helps you gain the momentum you will need in the long run to sustain your practice. The quality of your meditation is more significant than the length, as many meditation experts suggest.

3. Pick a convenient time and comfortable spot

Finding a quiet place away from noisy distractions is one of the best ways to meditate at home. Choose a time that is convenient for you. Since this time of day is generally peaceful and there are few interruptions, early morning is a perennial favorite time to meditate. With simple morning meditation exercises, you can also start your day.

You'll also need to find a comfortable position. There are other good options, although some meditators like sitting in the lotus position. As long as you feel relaxed and sit straight up, you can sit on a meditation pad, chair, or even a sofa. To find a place where your spine is aligned, do your best. Your neck and shoulders should be relaxed, and during the meditation session, your eyes may be half-open or shut.

4. Try a guided meditation

Directed meditation will bring a welcome structure to your practice because you're just starting. Mindworks App is a complete resource created and curated by globally recognized meditation experts that offers Guided Meditations, Mind Talks, inspiring Daily Cups, and much more. Choose from the guided meditations, have a seat, and enjoy the ride. To get you started, Mindworks provides a free trial period with everything you need.

5. Focus

Whatever type of meditation you choose, the present moment's awareness is essential. When you meditate, you train yourself to be mindful of whatever meditation object you have picked. There may be disturbances in the form of sounds, smells, feelings of pain, tension, scratching, etc. Moreover, the mind can create distractions all by itself: to-do lists, things you should have done or said, things you expect to do or say, feelings, daydreams... the list is endless.

One of the easiest ways to meditate at home is to concentrate on the rhythm of breathing to help the mind remain focused on the here and now. When you inhale and exhale, be very mindful of your breathing; use your breath as an anchor for your mind. Simply understand their presence and return to concentrating on the breath when those intrusive thoughts pop into your brain. Alternatively, as your meditation focus, you can use physical stimuli, sound, or a visual object. Forget about emptying the mind.' What meditation is all about is noticing and getting back.

6. Goodness

Trungram Gyalwa, a renowned Himalayan meditation master, teaches that compassion is a basic attribute that in all of us is hard-wired. Meditation allows one to regulate negative feelings (such as anger and envy) and reveal positive traits such as compassion and loving-kindness. Meditation gives us all the instruments we need to cultivate the goodness inside which there is already.

HOW TO MEDITATE EFFECTIVELY

Meditation is an approach to mental training, analogous to how fitness is an approach to body training. But there are also meditation methods, so how do you learn how to meditate? In the Buddhist tradition, the term "meditation" in the United States is similar to a word such as "sports." It's a family of things, not a single thing,' Richard J. Davidson, Ph.D., director of the University of Wisconsin neuroscience lab, told The New York Times. And different practices of meditation require various mental abilities.

It's incredibly hard for a beginner to sit for hours and think about nothing or have an "empty mind." We have some tools to help you through this process while you are only beginning to learn how to meditate best, such as a beginner meditation DVD or a brain-sensing headband. The best way to start meditating, in general, is by concentrating on the breath. Concentration is an example of one of the most popular approaches to meditation.

CONCENTRATION MEDITATION

Meditation on attention requires concentrating on a single point. This may include breathing, repeating a single word or mantra, looking at a candle flame, listening to a repeated gong, or counting a mala bead. Since it is difficult to concentrate the mind, a beginner might meditate for just a few minutes and then practice for longer durations.

Each time you find your mind wandering in this type of meditation, you simply refocus your consciousness on the chosen object of attention. You let them go rather than chasing random thoughts. Over this cycle, the ability to focus increases.

- Lower blood pressure
- Improved blood circulation
- Lower heart rate
- Less perspiration
- Slower respiratory rate

- Less anxiety
- Lower blood cortisol levels
- More feelings of well-being
- Less stress
- Deeper relaxation

Contemporary researchers are now investigating whether meditation's daily practice provides long-term benefits, noting positive effects among meditators on the brain and immune function. Nevertheless, it is worth repeating that the purpose of meditation is not to attain benefits. The goal of meditation is no goal, as an Eastern philosopher might say, to put it. It is only to be there.

The ultimate benefit of meditation in Buddhist philosophy is the liberation of the mind from attachment to things that it can not control, such as external conditions or strong internal emotions. No longer needlessly follows impulses or clings to experiences, the liberated or "enlightened" practitioner, but still retains a balanced mind and sense of inner peace.

HOW TO MEDITATE: SIMPLE MEDITATION FOR BEGINNERS

An outstanding introduction to meditation techniques is this meditation exercise.

1. Comfortably sit or lie. You may even wish to invest in a chair or cushion for meditation.

2. Your eyes close. When lying down, we consider using one of our Cooling Eye Masks or Restorative Eye Pillows.

3. Do not attempt to regulate your breath; just breathe naturally.

4. With each inhalation and exhalation, concentrate your attention on the breath and on how the body moves. Note the body's motion when you breathe. Watch your chest, your shoulders, your rib cage, and your belly. Without monitoring its speed or strength, simply concentrate your attention on your breath. Return your attention to your breath if your mind wanders.

For two to three minutes to start, continue this meditation practice, and then try it for longer periods.

Chapter 18: BEST WAYS TO MAINTAIN WEIGHT LOSS

Sadly, many individuals who lose weight end up gaining it back.

Only about 20 percent of overweight dieters end up losing weight effectively and holding it off in the long term.

Don't let this stop you, though. There are a variety of clinically validated ways to keep weight off, from exercise to stress management.

These 17 tactics may be exactly what you need to tip the numbers in your favor and keep your weight loss hard-won.

Why People Restore Weight

There are some common reasons why people gain back the weight they lose. They are often linked to irrational impulses and emotions of deprivation.

Restrictive diets: Drastic limits on calories can slow your metabolism and alter your appetite-regulating hormones, all of which lead to weight recovery.

Wrong mindset: You would be more likely to give up and regain the weight you lost if you think of a diet as a fast fix rather than a long-term approach to boost your health.

Lack of sustainable habits: Most diets are focused on willpower rather than on habits that you can integrate into your everyday life. Rather than lifestyle improvements, they concentrate on guidelines, which can deter you and avoid weight maintenance.

With criteria that are hard to keep up with, many diets are too restrictive. Additionally, before beginning a diet, many individuals do not have the correct mentality, leading to weight recovery.

1. Exercise Often

For weight management, daily exercise plays a significant role.

It will help you burn some extra calories and improve your metabolism, two variables required to maintain energy balance.

It means that you burn the same amount of calories you consume while you're in the energy balance. Consequently, the weight is more likely to remain the same.

Several studies have shown that people who do moderate physical exercise for at least 200 minutes a week (30 minutes a day) following weight loss are more likely to maintain weight. In certain cases, for good weight management, even greater levels of physical activity might be required. One research found that one hour of exercise a day is suitable for sustaining weight loss.

It is important to remember that when paired with other lifestyle improvements, including keeping to a balanced diet, exercise is the most beneficial for weight maintenance.

By helping balance your calories and calories expended, exercising for at least 30 minutes a day will encourage weight maintenance.

2. Try Eating Breakfast Every Day

For your weight loss goals, having breakfast will benefit you. Breakfast eaters prefer to usually have healthy habits, such as walking more and eating more fiber and micronutrients

Besides, eating breakfast is one of the most common habits recorded by people who are successful at sustaining weight loss.

One study found that 78 percent of 2,959 individuals who sustained a weight loss of 30 pounds (14 kg) for at least one year reported eating breakfast daily.

Nevertheless, while people who eat breakfast tend to be very good at sustaining weight loss, the evidence is mixed.

Research does not suggest that missing breakfast immediately leads to weight gain or worse eating habits.

Skipping breakfast can also help some people achieve their goals of weight loss and weight maintenance.

This may be one of the things that come down to the guy.

If you find that eating breakfast makes you stick to your objectives, you should certainly eat it. But if you don't want to eat breakfast or are not hungry in the morning, skipping it doesn't harm you.

Those eating breakfasts tend to usually have healthy habits, which may help them control their weight. Skipping breakfast, however, does not immediately lead to an increase in weight.

3. Eat Lots of Protein

You can control your weight by consuming a lot of protein because protein can help suppress appetite and encourage fullness.

Protein raises levels in the body of certain hormones that cause satiety and are important for weight control. It has also been shown that protein decreases hormone levels that enhance appetite.

The effect of protein on your hormones and fullness will automatically decrease the number of calories you eat each day, a significant factor in weight maintenance.

Also, for your body to break down, protein takes a large amount of energy. Eating it daily will also increase the number of calories you burn during the day.

Based on several studies, the effects of protein on metabolism and appetite tend to be most pronounced when around 30 percent of protein calories are consumed. On a 2,000 calorie diet, that's 150 grams of protein

Weight maintenance will benefit from protein by encouraging fullness, increasing metabolism, and reducing your overall calorie intake.

4. Weigh Yourself Regularly

A helpful method for weight management might be to track your weight by standing on the scale regularly. This is because it will make you conscious of your success and promote behavioral weight management.

Those weighing themselves will also consume fewer calories during the day, which helps to sustain weight loss.

On average, in one study, people who weighed themselves six days a week ate 300 fewer calories a day than those who tracked their weight less often.

A personal alternative is how much you weigh yourself. Others find it advantageous to weigh in regularly, while others measure their weight once or twice a week more effectively.

By keeping you mindful of your progress and habits, self-weighing will help weight management.

5. Be mindful of your carb intake

If you pay attention to the types and quantities of carbohydrates you consume, weight control can be easier to achieve.

It may be harmful to your weight-loss objectives to eat too many processed carbohydrates, such as white bread, white pasta, and fruit juices.

These foods, which are essential to encourage fullness, have been stripped of their natural fiber. Low-fiber diets are associated with weight gain and obesity.

It can also help you sustain your weight loss by limiting your carb intake overall. Many studies have shown that people who adopt low-carb diets following weight loss are more likely to hold the weight off in the long term, in some cases. Furthermore, people on low-carb diets are less likely to consume more calories than burn, which is important for weight maintenance.

Limiting your carbohydrate intake, particularly those that are processed, can help prevent weight recovery.

6. Lift Weights

A common side effect of weight loss is decreased muscle mass.

As losing muscle decreases your metabolism, it can limit your ability to hold the weight off, meaning you burn fewer calories during the day (34).

Doing any form of resistance training, such as weight lifting, can help avoid this muscle loss and, in turn, sustain or even increase your metabolic rate.

Studies show that by retaining muscle mass, those who lift weights after weight loss are more likely to hold weight off It is recommended to participate in strength training at least twice a week to obtain these benefits. For optimum performance, your training regimen should work for all muscle groups.

Maintaining your muscle mass, which is vital to maintain a healthy metabolism, lifting weights at least twice a week will help with weight maintenance.

7. Be Prepared for Setbacks

Setbacks on your weight maintenance trip are unavoidable. When you give in to an unhealthy craving or miss a workout, there can be occasions.

However, the occasional slip-up does not mean that you can throw your goals out of the window. Simply move on with better options and follow through.

It can also help prepare for circumstances that you know would make healthy eating difficult, such as an upcoming holiday or vacation, in advance.

Since losing weight, you may face a setback or two. By planning and getting back on track right away, you will overcome setbacks.

8. Stick to your schedule Long All Week (Even on Weekends)

Eating well on weekdays and cheating on weekends is one habit that also contributes to weight recovery.

This mentality also causes individuals to binge on fast food, which can offset attempts to control weight.

You could recover more weight than you lost in the first place if it becomes a daily habit.

Alternatively, evidence suggests that those who follow a healthy eating routine all during the week are more likely to achieve long-term weight loss.

One study found that weekly consistency made people nearly twice as likely over a year to keep their weight within five pounds (2.2 kg), compared to those who allowed more flexibility on weekends

When you stick to your healthy eating habits all week long, good weight loss is easicr to achieve, even on weekends.

9. Remain hydrated

For a few purposes, drinking water is good for weight maintenance.

First, if you drink a glass or two before meals, it encourages fullness and will help you keep your calorie intake in check.

In one study, relative to people who didn't drink water, those who drank water before consuming a meal had a 13 percent reduction in calorie intake.

Also, drinking water has been shown to increase the number of calories you burn during the day slightly.

Drinking water will frequently stimulate fullness and increase your metabolism, both of which are significant weight loss factors.

10. Get Enough Sleep

Having enough sleep strongly impacts weight management.

In truth, sleep deprivation appears to be a significant risk factor in adults for weight gain and may interfere with weight maintenance.

This is partly because insufficient sleep contributes to higher ghrelin levels, which is referred to as the hormone of hunger. After all, it raises appetite.

Also, poor sleepers appear to have lower levels of leptin, a hormone essential for regulating appetite.

Also, those who sleep for short periods are exhausted and therefore less driven to make healthy food decisions and exercise.

If you don't have enough time, find a way to change your sleeping patterns. For weight management and good wellbeing, sleeping for at least seven hours a night is optimum.

Keeping your energy levels up and hormones under the balance, sleeping for a reasonable amount of time will help with weight maintenance.

11. Control Stress Levels

A significant part of maintaining your weight is handling stress.

In fact, by increasing the cortisol levels, which is a hormone released in response to stress, high levels of stress may lead to weight recovery.

Higher levels of belly fat are associated with chronically elevated cortisol and increased appetite and food intake.

Stress, which is when you eat even when you're not hungry, is also a common cause for impulsive eating.

Fortunately, to combat tension, there are many things you can do, including exercise, yoga, and meditation.

To maintain your weight, it is important to keep stress levels under control, as excess stress can increase the risk of weight gain by stimulating your appetite.

12. Find a Support System

Maintaining your weight goals alone can be challenging.

One solution is to find a support group that can keep you accountable and probably works with you in your healthier lifestyle to solve this.

A few studies have shown that it can be beneficial for weight control to have a buddy to follow your goals, particularly if that individual is a partner or spouse with similar healthy habits.

One of these studies analyzed the health habits of over 3,000 couples and found that the other was more likely to follow their example when one partner participated in a healthy habit, such as exercise.

Involving a partner or spouse in your healthy lifestyle may increase the chance that your weight loss will be maintained.

13. Track Your Food Intake

Many who monitor their food intake may be more likely to sustain their weight loss in a journal, online food tracker, or app.

Food trackers are useful because they improve how much you eat since they also offer detailed details on how many calories and nutrients you consume.

Also, several food monitoring apps allow you to record exercise, so you can make sure you get the amount you need to maintain your weight.

Here are some examples of websites and applications for calorie counting.

By making you aware of how many calories and nutrients you eat, logging your food intake from day to day can help you maintain your weight loss.

14. Eat Plenty of Vegetables

Many studies relate high consumption of vegetables to better control of weight.

Vegetables are low in calories, to start with. Without piling on weight, you can eat huge portions while still eating an incredible amount of nutrients.

Vegetables are also high in fiber, which increases feelings of fullness and may minimize the number of calories you consume during the day automatically.

Aim to eat a serving or two of vegetables at any meal for these weight management advantages.

Vegetables have a high fiber content and are low in calories. For weight management, both of these properties may be helpful.

15. Be Consistent

Consistency is important for weight loss.

It is best to stick with your new balanced diet and lifestyle for good instead of on-and-off dieting, ending with going back to old habits.

While it can at first seem daunting to embrace a new way of life, making healthier choices can become second nature as you get used to them.

Your healthy lifestyle would be effortless, making it far easier for you to control your weight.

Instead of going back to your old lifestyle, sustaining weight loss is easy when you are consistent with your new healthy habits.

16. Practice Mindful Eating

Mindful eating is the activity during the eating process of listening to internal appetite signs and paying complete attention.

It includes eating slowly, without distractions, and thoroughly chewing the food so you can savor your meal's aroma and taste.

You are more likely to stop eating when you are full when you eat this way. It can be hard to notice fullness if you eat when distracted, and you can end up overeating

Research shows that mindful eating helps to maintain weight by targeting habits that are often related to weight gain, such as emotional eating

What's more, without counting calories, those who eat carefully will control their weight

For weight management, mindful eating is helpful because it makes you accept fullness and avoid harmful habits that normally contribute to weight gain.

17. Make Sustainable Changes to Your Lifestyle

Many individuals struggle to control their weight because restrictive diets are practiced that are not practical in the long term.

They end up feeling deprived, which also leads to a greater weight gain than they lost in the first place until they return to eating normally.

It is down to make sustainable improvements to your diet to maintain weight loss.

For everybody, this looks different, but ultimately it means not being too rigid, remaining consistent, and making healthy decisions as much as possible.

When you make sustainable lifestyle changes, it is easier to maintain weight loss than following the unrealistic guidelines that many weight-loss diets concentrate on.

About the bottom line

Diets may be restrictive and impractical, often leading to a recovery of weight.

There are, however, several quick improvements that you can make to the habits that are easy to adhere to and can help you sustain your long-term weight loss.

You will learn during your journey that managing your weight requires far more than what you eat. A function is also played by exercise, sleep, and mental wellbeing.

If you simply follow a new lifestyle, rather than going on and off weight-loss diets, weight management can be effortless.

Chapter 19: THE CONNECTION BETWEEN SLEEP AND WEIGHT

The amount of time Americans spend sleeping has gradually decreased over the past few decades, as has the self-reported importance of that sleep. The average body mass index (BMI) of Americans rose for most of the same period, representing a trend towards higher body weights and elevated rates of obesity.

Many researchers started hypothesizing about possible correlations between weight and sleep in response to these patterns. Several studies have shown that limited sleep and poor sleep quality can lead to metabolic disorders, weight gain, and an increased risk of obesity and other chronic health problems.

Although the medical community continues to question the exact essence of this relationship, the latest study points to a strong connection between good sleep and healthy body weight.

A lot remains to be learned about the nuanced details of how sleep and weight are related. Several theories provide avenues for further study, hoping that strengthening our understanding of the relationship between weight and sleep would lead to decreased obesity and improved weight loss methods.

Will sleep deprivation raise your appetite?

How sleep influences appetite is one popular theory about the relationship between weight and sleep. While we sometimes think of appetite as simply a matter of grumbling in the stomach, neurotransmitters, which are chemical messengers that enable neurons (nerve cells) to communicate with each other, actually regulate it.

It is known that the neurotransmitters ghrelin and leptin are central to appetite. Ghrelin promotes hunger, and leptin leads to feeling full. Throughout the day, the body gradually raises and decreases these neurotransmitters' levels, suggesting the need to eat calories.

A lack of sleep may influence the control of these neurotransmitters by the body. In one study, relative to those who got 10 hours of sleep, men who got 4 hours of sleep had increased ghrelin and decreased leptin. In people who are sleep deprived, this dysregulation of ghrelin and leptin can lead to increased appetite and diminished fullness feelings. Furthermore, some studies have also shown that food preferences are influenced by sleep deprivation. Sleep-deprived people prefer to select foods that are high in calories and carbohydrates.

The body's endocannabinoid system5 and orexin6, a neurotransmitter targeted by certain sleep aids, are other theories about the connection between sleep and increased appetite.

Many researchers believe that the relationship between sleep and neurotransmitter dysregulation is complicated and more studies are needed to further understand the neurobiological relationship.

Does Metabolism Improve Sleep?

Metabolism7 is a chemical mechanism in which the body transforms the energy required to live into what we eat and drink. Metabolism is part of all of our collective practices, from breathing to exercise and everything in between. Although activities like exercise can increase metabolism temporarily, sleep can't8. Metabolism slows down by about 15 percent during sleep, reaching its lowest level by 9 in the morning.

Several studies have shown that sleep deficiency typically contributes to metabolic dysregulation (whether due to self-induction, insomnia, untreated sleep apnea, or other sleep disorders). Elevated oxidative stress, glucose (blood sugar) intolerance (a precursor to diabetes), and insulin resistance are associated with poor sleep. Extra time spent awake can increase the chances of eating11, and less sleep can interfere with circadian rhythms, contributing to weight gain12.

How is Sleep Related to Physical Activity?

Losing sleep can result in less energy for physical activity and exercise. Feeling exhausted can also do sports and exercise less safe, especially weightlifting activities and those requiring balance. While researchers are still trying to understand this connection,13 it is well known that to maintain weight loss and good health, exercise is important.

Getting regular exercise can improve sleep quality, especially if natural light is involved in the exercise. Although even taking a short walk during the day will help boost sleep, there can be a more drastic effect on more activity. It can increase daytime concentration and decrease daytime sleepiness by engaging in at least 150 minutes of moderate-intensity or 75 minutes of high-intensity exercise per week.

Obesity and Sleep

The correlation between not getting enough sleep and an increased risk of obesity is well-established in children and adolescents, although this link's explanation is still being debated. As discussed earlier, insufficient sleep in children can lead to metabolic disturbances, missing breakfast in the morning, and increased consumption of sweet, salty, fatty, and starchy foods15.

In adults, the study is less apparent. Although a broad review of past research shows that individuals who get less than 6 hours of sleep at night are more likely to be diagnosed as obese,16, it is difficult to determine cause and effect for these studies. Obesity itself, including sleep apnea and depression, may raise the risk of having disorders that interfere with sleep. In these studies, it is not clear whether having less sleep is the cause of obesity, whether obesity causes the participants to get less sleep, or maybe both. While more studies are needed to understand this correlation, when treating obesity in adults, experts recommend improving the quality of sleep.

Sleep During Weight Loss

A significant part of a successful weight loss strategy is to get enough good-quality sleep. Research has shown, most significantly, that losing sleep while dieting will reduce the number of weight lost17 and promote overeating.

TIPS FOR SLEEP QUALITY DURING WEIGHT LOSS

Several ways can be changed. Here are a few tips focused on studies to sleep easier while you're trying to lose weight:

Keep a daily sleep schedule: Major fluctuations in your sleep schedule or trying to catch up on sleep after a week of late nights can cause metabolic changes and decrease insulin sensitivity, making it easier to increase blood sugar.

Sleep in a dark room: artificial light exposure during sleep, such as a TV or bedside lamp, is associated with an increased risk of gaining weight and obesity.

Do not eat right before bed: Eating late can decrease the effectiveness of attempts to lose weight.

Stress reduction: Constant stress can lead to poor sleep and weight gain in many ways, including eating to deal with adverse emotions.

Be an Early Bird: People with late bedtimes can eat more calories and have a higher chance of gaining weight. Early birds, relative to night owls24, may be more likely to sustain weight loss.

Keeping a healthy relationship with your body

A personal decision best taken with your doctor's advice is to determine whether you should try to change your body weight. Do not take at face value all the health and weight loss data you read online25. Weight loss is not ideal for all and does not necessarily indicate improved health. Bear in mind that wellness is a lifelong process that requires healthy behaviors and a healthy link with your body. The National Institutes of Health provides a helpful resource for selecting a healthy weight loss program if you consider weight loss.

17 SNEAKY WAYS TO LOSE WEIGHT IN YOUR SLEEP

Yesterday, how many meals did you eat?

But you answered the above question, though; the chances are that you probably eat much more often than you remember. According to a report at The Salk Institute, most of us now cram multiple mini-meals into our daily meals. And the longer we sit up, the more we eat calories.

The researchers speculated that the best way to minimize calorie intake could be simply to get more sleep, so they asked people who ate every day for 14 hours to reduce their grazing time to no more than 11 hours a day and to sleep more than once a day. Subjects lost an average of 3.5% of their excess body weight after 16 weeks, only by going to bed earlier.

That means there are just a few quick tweaks to your p.m. Severe weight loss success can be inferred by routine. So open your eyes: here are suggestions to fail when you sleep that is science-backed. And while you are awake, make sure that you try these 21 Best Safe Cooking Hacks of All Time to keep you on board with your goals for weight loss!

Try your sleep switch

Sheep, don't count, eat lamb! Or even better, a bit of turkey. Effective sleep-inducing effects were shown by tryptophan, an amino acid found in most meats. Research published in The Journal of Nervous and Mental Illness among "mild" insomniacs found that only 1/4 gram was adequate to dramatically increase hours of a deep sleep, around what you would find in a skinless chicken drumstick or three ounces of lean turkey meat. And that could translate into quick weight loss.

"Any tryptophan-containing food, which includes nuts, chicken, fish, lentils, and eggs, can help usher in sleepyhead syndrome," says Julia Falamas, coach of New York's Crossfit Spot Barbell. "If you're the type who can't sleep on an empty stomach, a healthy source of fat like avocado or nut butter can help stave off hunger while providing restorative properties," she adds.

2 Schedule tea time

"There is something about the ritual of sitting down to a soothing cup of tea that tells your brain to slow down and relax," Falamas says. "Some of the best teas for sleep are chamomile, peppermint, lavender, and valerian, which does have some sedative properties."

3 At lunch, eat whole grains.

Before bed, you know how to stop huge meals, coffee, colas, and alcohol, but did you know it's better to eat your complex carbohydrates for lunch, not for dinner? "Serotonin converts to melatonin in your stage 3 REM sleep, and serotonin is sourced from whole-grain complex carbohydrates. So you don't need to have carbs before bed to sleep, just have them at some point through the day," says Cat Smiley, owner of Whistler Fitness Vacations, a women's weight loss retreat. Also, "about 20 grams of insoluble fiber is important to enable you to sleep, so aim to eat that daily, and you'll ensure you can convert enough serotonin to sleep well." to achieve your daily fiber target.

4 If you eat at night, keep it small
Although you should not go to bed hungry (which poses problems with sleep), you shouldn't hit the sack fully stuffed, either. Your body works to digest it well into the night when you consume a big meal before bed. And if your body is still worked up, so are you. The later you fall asleep, the less rest you get, and you wake up feeling groggy and more likely to reach for things that are rich in calories.
Try to keep portions approximately the same as your breakfast and lunch instead of eating a monster meal for dinner, particularly if you eat dinner later. "You want to eat your last meal at least an hour or two before going to bed," says Isabel Smith, MS, RD, CDN.
5 Better still, set strict hours for kitchens
According to a study in the journal Cell Metabolism, nighttime fasting, aka closing the kitchen early, can help you lose more weight, even if you eat more food during the day. Experiment with the 8 p.m. closure of the kitchen Skipping and breakfast.
6 Try a protein shake
Protein shake lady - how to lose weight overnight
Shutterstock Shutterstock

According to one Florida State University report, getting a protein shake before hitting the sack can boost your metabolism. Researchers found that the next morning, men who consumed an evening snack containing 30 grams of protein had a higher resting metabolic rate than when they didn't eat something. Protein is more thermogenic than carbs or fat, ensuring that more calories are consumed by the body digesting it.

Using vegan protein powder that will give you the same benefits of fat-burning, hunger-squelching, muscle-building, without whey-based bloating.

7 Relax with meditation, breathing, or stretching

Because of yoga's emphasis on breathing and meditation, striking some poses before bed can have a powerful effect on sleep quality. "Yoga offers a variety of benefits, from increased flexibility and strength to a calmer mind," says Mark Balfe-Taylor, TruFusion's yoga owner. He suggests The Posture of the Deaf Man.

It can calm the nervous system, release the shoulders and neck, and allows you to concentrate inward, block stress, and relax; most importantly, "It can calm the nervous system, release the shoulders and neck, and, most importantly, allows you to focus inward, block out stress and relax,"

8 Let in the cold

Striking new research published in the journal Diabetes indicates that it can help us attack belly fat as we sleep by simply blasting the air conditioner or turning down the winter heat. Colder temperatures subtly increase the productivity of our fat brown stores. Fat helps you warm by helping you burn the fat contained in your stomach. In bedrooms with different temperatures, participants spent a few weeks sleeping: a neutral 75 degrees, a mild 66 degrees, and a balmy 81 degrees. After sleeping at 66 degrees for four weeks, the subjects nearly doubled their amount of brown fat. (And yes, it means that they have lost belly fat.)

9 Throw out the night light

According to a recent study published in the American Journal of Epidemiology, exposure to light at night does not only disrupt your chances of a great night's sleep, but it may also result in weight gain. Research participants sleeping in the darkest rooms were 21% less likely than those sleeping in the lightest rooms to be obese.

That leads us to our next trick of sleep-slimming...

10 Hide the iPad

Research indicates that, particularly among kids, the more electronics we bring into the bedroom, the fatter we get. Research in the journal Pediatric Obesity found that kids who bask in a TV or computer's nighttime glow don't get enough rest and suffer from bad lifestyle habits. Researchers found that students with access to one electronic device were 1.47 times as likely as children with no devices in the bedroom to be overweight. That increased for children with three devices to 2.57 times.

Bottom line: In the living room, leave your iPad. Maybe your partner will thank you, too.

11 Turn off the TV

Did you know that slim people watch less television? A recent review of JAMA studies showed that the risk of developing diabetes, developing heart disease, and early death increased by 20, 15, and 13 percent, respectively, for every two hours spent watching TV. Scientists are still working out why sitting is so dangerous to health, but one obvious and partial reason is that the less we move, the less fuel we need; the blood sugar excess fills the bloodstream and leads to diabetes and other risks associated with weight.

With these best-ever diet tips, find out how only a few other basic tweaks will help you lose up to 4 inches from your waist easily!

12 Blackout with blackout shades

When it comes to falling asleep, light-blocking curtains make a massive difference. Even if you think you're immune to such instinctive cues, external light makes it harder for your mind to shut down. When light is present, melatonin, the hormone involved in putting the body to sleep, is compromised.

"Darken your room so that going to bed, even early, feels natural," Smiley says.

13 Take a hot shower

If you usually bathe in the morning, listen up. "A hot shower is great for ensuring a good night's sleep because it can help relieve tension and relax sore muscles. Additionally, it can increase the level of oxytocin—a 'love' hormone released by your brain—which can be very soothing," Falamas says. The heat from the shower also boosts your body temperature, resulting in a rapid drop in temperature as you get out and towel off, a dip that allows your whole system to relax. Also, a hot bath will have the same effect.

14 Skip the chocolate

Don't get us wrong; chocolate is what we do. In fact, because of its high concentration of antioxidants and stress-busting capacity, any bar that contains at least 70 percent cacao is one of our favorite low-sugar snacks or desserts. Unfortunately, this chocolate might be the reason you can't fall asleep if you eat it too late. According to Market Lab research, dark chocolate contains caffeine-approximately 40 to 50 mg of caffeine per 40-gram serving, which may keep the body from shutting down when you want it to if you are responsive to the compound.

Chocolate bars have varying caffeine levels, but there are about 79 milligrams in a typical two-ounce, 70 percent dark chocolate bar. An eight-ounce cup of coffee contains around 145 milligrams, for reference. Try these filling, guilt-free weight loss snacks for a new late-night indulgence!

15 Do not indulge yourself in a nightcap

Thanks to its resveratrol, a plant compound that has been correlated with heart-healthy benefits, wine are our favorite "healthy" alcoholic drink. However, further research needs to be done, according to a study published in the journal Nutrients. However, according to Smith, the evening glass of wine is often considered a high-sugar beverage. Drinking too much will impair your snoozing ability. It may feel like that nightly glass of wine relaxes you and makes you fall asleep quicker. Still, it keeps your body from completely indulging in its REM (Rapid Eye Movement) period, which is when sleep and dreaming are truly restful.

To stop sleep disturbance, enjoy a glass earlier in the night, around two hours before bedtime, and close the home bar after one or two glasses, tops.

16 Have more sex

Will you like to sleep better and lose some weight? Get sex even more. New research published in the Journal of Sexual Medicine shows that their sexual appetite increased correspondingly with every extra hour of sleep women got. And separate studies by Dr. Michele Lastella, an Adelaide sleep expert, found that the more sex you get, the better you sleep and the more weight you lose.

17 On a pillow splurge

Some appliances are complete ripoffs when it comes to a better night's sleep (like those as-seen-on-TV anti-snoring gadgets), but it is important to invest in the right pillow. "Buying an orthopedic pillow keeps your neck aligned. You'll wake up in the morning with no neck pain," Smiley says.

Chapter 20: TIPS FOR LOSING WEIGHT THAT is TRULY EVIDENCE-BASED

1. Water drinking, particularly before meals
Drinking water is also believed to be able to help with weight loss, and that is real.
Over 1-1.5 hours, drinking water will increase your metabolism by 24-30 percent, helping you consume a few more calories.
One study found that drinking half an hour before meals with half a liter (17 ounces) of water helped dieters consume fewer calories and lose 44 percent more weight than those who did not drink water.
2. For Breakfast, Eat Eggs
There can be all kinds of advantages to eating whole eggs, like helping you lose weight.
Studies show that substituting eggs for a grain-based breakfast will help you consume fewer calories for the next 36 hours and lose more body fat and weight.
That's perfect if you don't eat eggs. Any breakfast source of quality protein should do the trick.
3. Drink your coffee (Preferably Black)
Coffee has been demonized unfairly. Quality coffee is filled with antioxidants and can have many benefits for your well-being.
Studies show that coffee caffeine can improve metabolism by 3-11% and increase fat burning by 10-29%.
Only make sure your coffee doesn't add a lot of sugar or other high-calorie ingredients. That will eliminate any advantages.
At your nearest grocery store, as well as online, you can shop for coffee.

4. Have a drink of Green Tea

Green tea, like coffee, also has many advantages, one of them being weight loss.

Although green tea contains small amounts of caffeine, it is loaded with potent antioxidants called catechins, which are thought to improve fat burning synergistically with caffeine. Although the evidence is mixed, many studies show that green tea can help you lose weight (either as a drink or a supplement of green tea extract).

At most pharmacies, health stores, grocery stores, and online, green tea is available.

5. Try the Fasting Intermittent

A common eating pattern in which people alternate between periods of fasting and eating is intermittent fasting.

Short-term studies show that intermittent fasting is as effective as continuous calorie restriction for weight loss. Also, the loss of muscle mass usually associated with low-calorie diets can be minimized. However, before any stronger statements can be made, higher-quality studies are needed.

6. Take a supplement with Glucomannan

In many studies, a fiber called glucomannan has been related to weight loss.

This fiber source absorbs water and stays for a while in your stomach, making you feel fuller and helping you consume fewer calories.

Studies indicate that people who use glucomannan supplements lose a little more weight than those who do not. Glucomannan supplements can be found not only in vitamin shops and pharmacies but also online.

7. Cut Back on Added Sugar

One of the worst ingredients in the western diet is added sugar. Many individuals eat way too much.

Studies show that intake of sugar (and high-fructose corn syrup) is closely related to an increased risk of obesity and conditions such as type 2 diabetes and heart disease.

Cut down on added sugar if you want to lose weight. Just be sure to read labels since sugar can also be loaded with so-called health foods.

8. Eat Less Refined Carbs

Sugar and grains that have been deprived of their fibrous, nutritious portions contain processed carbohydrates. These include pasta and white bread.

Studies show that refined carbs can easily spike blood sugar, leading a few hours later to hunger, cravings, and increased food intake. Eating processed carbohydrates is closely correlated with obesity.

Be sure to feed them with their natural fiber if you're going to eat carbs.

9. Go on a Diet Low-Carb

Then consider going all the way and sticking to a low-carb diet if you want to get all carb restriction advantages.

Several studies indicate that such a regimen will help you lose 2-3 times as much weight as a regular low-fat diet while improving your health as well.

10. Smaller Plates Use

Using smaller plates has been shown to help certain individuals consume fewer calories automatically.

The plate-size effect doesn't seem to affect anyone, however. It seems like those who are overweight are more affected.

11. Exercise Portion Control or Calories Count

For obvious purposes, portion control-just eating less-or counting calories may be beneficial.

Some studies show that it can help you lose weight by keeping a food diary or taking pictures of your meals. Something that enhances your knowledge of what you consume may be advantageous.

12. If you get hungry, keep healthy food around in case you

If you become overly hungry, having nutritious food nearby will help prevent you from consuming something unhealthy. Whole fruits, nuts, baby carrots, milk, and hard-boiled eggs are conveniently portable and easy to prepare.

13. Take supplements with probiotics

It has been shown that taking probiotic supplements containing bacteria from the subfamily of Lactobacillus decreases fat mass.

The same doesn't apply to all species of Lactobacillus, however. Some research has linked L. Acidophilus with a gain in weight.

At many grocery stores, as well as online, you can shop for probiotic supplements.

14. Eat spicy foods

There is capsaicin in chili peppers, a spicy compound that can improve your metabolism and slightly reduce your appetite.

People can, however, grow immunity over time to the effects of capsaicin, which may limit its long-term efficacy.

15. Do cardiovascular exercises

An excellent way to lose calories and improve your physical and mental health is to do aerobic exercise (cardio).

The loss of belly fat, the unhealthy fat that tends to build up around your organs and cause metabolic disease, seems to be especially effective.

16. Lift Weights

One of the worst side effects of dieting also referred to as starvation mode, is that it appears to cause muscle loss and metabolic slowing.

Any type of resistance exercise, such as lifting weights, is the best way to avoid this. Research shows that weight lifting will help keep the metabolism up and avoid the loss of important muscle mass.

It's essential, of course, not just to lose weight; you also want to build muscle. For a toned body, resistance training is important.

17. Eat More Fiber

For weight loss, fiber is often recommended.

While there is mixed evidence, some studies show that fiber (especially viscous fiber) can increase satiety and help you manage your weight over the long term.

18. Eat More Fruit and Vegetables

There are many properties in vegetables and fruits that make them successful for weight loss.

There are few calories in them, but a lot of fiber. Their high content of water gives them a low density of energy, making them very complete.

Studies indicate that individuals who eat fruits and vegetables appear to weigh less.

Also, these foods are very healthy, so your health needs to eat them.

19. Take Good Sleep

Sleep is highly underrated, but it can be just as important as healthy eating and exercise.

Studies indicate that poor sleep is one of the highest risk factors for obesity. It is associated with an increased risk of obesity in children by 89 percent and adults by 55 percent.

20. Beat your addiction to food

A new study showed that 19.9 percent of North American and European individuals meet the food addiction criterion.

You can suffer from addiction if you have overpowering cravings and can't seem to curb your eating no matter how hard you try.

Seek clinical assistance in this instance. It's almost impossible to try to lose weight without first fighting against food addiction.

21. Eat More Protein

The single most significant nutrient for losing weight is protein.

It has been shown that eating a high-protein diet improves your metabolism by 80-100 calories a day while shaving 441 calories a day off your diet.

One research also found that consuming 25% of your daily calories as protein decreased repetitive food thoughts by 60% while reducing in half the appetite for late-night snacking.

One of the simplest and most effective ways to lose weight is to easily add protein to your diet.

22. Supplement With Whey Protein

If you struggle to get sufficient protein in your diet, it may help take a supplement, such as protein powder.

One study showed that replacing some of your calories with whey protein while increasing muscle mass can cause weight loss of about 8 pounds over time.

Whey protein is available online and at most health stores.

23. Don't Do Sugary Drinks, Including Soda and Fruit Juice

Sugar is bad, but sugar is even worse in liquid form. Studies show that the single most fattening aspect of the modern diet may be calories from liquid sugar.

For example, one study showed that sugar-sweetened beverages for each daily serving are linked to a 60% increased risk of obesity in children.

Keep in mind that this also applies to fruit juice, which, like a soft drink like Coke, contains a similar sugar amount.

Eat whole fruit, but entirely restrict or avoid fruit juice.

24. Eat whole foods, single-ingredient (Real Food)

If you want to be a leaner, healthier person, eating whole, single-ingredient foods are one of the best things you can do for yourself.

Naturally, these foods are filling, and if the majority of your diet is based on them, it is very hard to gain weight.

25. Don't Diet — Eat Healthy Instead

One of the biggest diet problems is that they seldom work in the long term.

People who diet tend to gain more weight over time if anything and studies demonstrate that dieting is a consistent predictor of future weight gain.

Try to become a healthier, happier, and fitter individual instead of going on a diet. Instead of depriving your body, focus on nourishing it.

Then weight loss should naturally follow.

26. Chew More Slowly

It may take a while for your brain to register that you have had enough to eat. Some studies show that chewing more slowly can help you eat fewer calories and boost weight loss-related hormones.

Consider chewing your food more carefully, too. Studies show that increased chewing may decrease a meal's intake of calories.

These practices are a component of mindful eating, helping you slow down your consumption of food and pay attention to each bite.

Various techniques can help your weight loss goals.

Some of the tips above are purely nutritional, including eating more protein or cutting back on added sugar.

Others are more lifestyle-based, like improving sleep quality or adding a workout routine. Chewing more slowly, for instance, is one step you can take to establish conscious eating.

You'll be well on your way to your weight loss goals if you implement a handful of these tips.

Chapter 21: FREQUENTLY ASKED QUESTIONS ABOUT HYPNOSIS

Q: What is hypnosis?

A: That's a tough question to respond to quickly and accurately. Some say it is an altered state of consciousness,' but because there is currently no agreed concept of consciousness, this argument can go around in circles. When we talk about hypnosis, we typically mean either the calm, concentrated, and absorbed feelings associated with a 'trance state' (although some people dislike the term trance), we tend to be talking about the interesting things people can do when hypnotized - these are the results of 'suggestion.'

Q: Is hypnosis real?

A: Yes, in a nutshell. Hypnotic suggestions can change people's perceptions and sensations, and beliefs. Hypnotic suggestions, for example, may be used to cause vivid hallucinations or improve pain perception. Hypnosis and hypnotic suggestions change how the brain processes information, according to studies that measure brain activity. Randomized controlled clinical trials have indicated that hypnosis can be an effective treatment for pain and an effective part of treatments for other conditions. Although it is indeed very easy to 'fake' a hypnotic response, there are also real observable results.

Q: Can anyone be hypnotized?
A: Yeah, anyone can be hypnotized to an extent - some more than others. A hypnotic susceptibility scale may be used to determine hypnosis susceptibility. People are usually graded as 'highs, "mediums,' or 'lows' by researchers. Around 80% of people fall into the medium category, which means they are prone to many of the effects of hypnotic suggestion and are likely to benefit from its therapeutic application if necessary. Approximately 10 percent of the population is considered highly hypnotizable, which implies they are easily hypnotized and may undergo drastic sensation and perception changes. Approximately 10% are rated as 'low,' indicating they have not reacted well to hypnosis (although some skills programs aim to increase hypnosis susceptibility).
Some clinicians, notably Milton Erickson, claim that everyone can be hypnotized but that the hypnotist must change their style or content. However, because the only way to test suggestibility is to look at how people react to suggestions, and because suggestibility is rarely tested in clinical settings, it's difficult to find any evidence to support this assertion.

Q: Can hypnotisability be modified?

A: Training programs have been developed to enhance participants' responses to suggestibility tests. Some researchers claim that the increase caused by this approach is merely the result of participants being motivated to respond without actually experiencing their response as involuntary (a criterion set by Weitzenhoffer as a "true" response to suggestion). On the other hand, other scholars claim that such 'educated high suggestible' participants' subjective responses are indistinguishable from those who are 'naturally high suggestible' without training. Some drugs have also been found to make people more suggestible.

Q: Is hypnosis dangerous?
A: Hypnosis isn't in itself a dangerous procedure, but there are worries that if it is not used correctly, it could have harmful side effects — the dangers of hypnosis (for example, participants may experience a mild headache).

Q: Can hypnosis make me do things I don't want to do?
A: No, you can't be compelled to do anything you don't want to do in hypnosis. In hypnosis, you maintain control over your ability to act on suggestions, though if you do allow yourself to act on a suggestion, the results can seem to occur on their own.

Orne and Evans performed a study to see if they could make hypnotized subjects do things like throwing a jar of acid in the face of a research assistant (the jar didn't contain acid for safety purposes, but the subjects in the experiment were unaware of this). They discovered that while 5 out of 6 high hypnotizable participants threw the 'acid,' 6 out of 6 low hypnotizable participants who were asked to mimic being in hypnosis also threw the 'acid.' This experiment reveals that it isn't something special about being in hypnosis that causes people to participate in antisocial acts, but rather the social situation in which the experiment was performed. The experiment's rationale is that if you can get people to perform antisocial actions without hypnosis (the low hypnotizables who were asked to pretend), you don't need hypnosis to justify what they're doing.

Q: Is hypnosis like sleep?
A: The answer is no. Hypnosis comes from the Greek god of sleep. Hypnos studies have shown that hypnosis and sleep are not the same things. While there are distinct brain activity patterns associated with sleep, hypnosis has not been shown in brain activity studies. Hypnosis may appear to observers to be similar to sleep because calming suggestions are often considered part of a hypnotic routine. Still, hypnotized people are in a state more akin to wakefulness (and hypnosis has also been induced in individuals riding exercise bicycles - so-called 'active alert' hypnosis).

Q: What does hypnosis feel like?

A: The answer is that hypnosis is likely to feel different for every individual. People generally equate hypnosis with a feeling of calm and many hypnotists (researchers and clinicians) use relaxation procedures. Different individuals have different bodily responses to relaxation instructions; some feel heavy, while others feel light, almost as though they are floating. Mentally, people respond in all sorts of ways. People often report feeling deeply concentrated or absorbed, often without even noticing it. People may have very vivid creative experiences when imagery instructions are used regularly; many people report feeling "as if they were there.

Q: Can I get 'stuck' in hypnosis?
A: There is no proof that someone may become stuck in hypnosis. The worst that can happen is that you fall asleep and wake up unhypnotized! Orne and Evans performed a well-known experiment in which participants were hypnotized. The experimenter left the room under the guise of needing to attend to a problem; the participant was then observed (without his knowledge) to see what happened.

Q: What conditions can hypnosis treat?
 A: Hypnosis is not a treatment in its own right, but when done by a trained doctor, or psychologist, it may help with several problems, including pain, anxiety
conditions (including panic attacks, phobia, and PTSD), irritable bowel syndrome, depression, and more.

Q: I'd like hypnosis to be part of my treatment; who can I see?

A: Hypnosis and psychotherapy are regulated differently in various countries, and in many countries, no special training is needed to call oneself a "hypnotherapist." According to the International Society of Hypnosis, only practitioners who are already trained in a clinical discipline (such as medicine, psychology, psychotherapy, or dentistry) should use hypnosis. To quote Martin Orne: "If someone isn't qualified to treat something without hypnosis, they aren't qualified to treat anything with hypnosis, either. You start by searching for a professional certificate on the wall — physician, dentist, clinical psychologist, or whatever. Then you look for the certificate of hypnosis."

Q: Is NLP like hypnosis?
A: Neuro-linguistic programming, or NLP, is a series of techniques aimed at fostering personal development. Some of these methods were developed by prominent hypnotherapists, most notably Milton Erickson. NLP is not a part of conventional academic psychology because it has not been scientifically tested. Skeptic, the skeptic's dictionary, has an excellent account of NLP.

Q: Are some words more suggestive than others?
When using hypnosis, it's important to use language carefully, but it's difficult to tell whether one word is more suggestive than another. It is now widely accepted that a person's ability to react to suggestion is determined more by their characteristics (suggestibility, absorption, and willingness) than by the hypnotist's authority or power. A clinician's style of hypnosis can vary from direct/authoritarian ("when I click my fingers you will feel ... ") to indirect/permissive ("as I continue to speak you might start to realize that the feeling becomes..."), and Milton Erickson's followers popularized indirect suggestion.
Experiments to compare the effects of these two forms of suggestions have been performed, but the results do not allow us to conclude that one is more effective.

Q: Can hypnosis help me to stop drinking alcohol?
A: There isn't much evidence that hypnosis is an effective alcoholism treatment. Nash and Benham note in a study that hypnosis does not function well for drug and alcohol addiction and two studies that I can find that compare hypnosis (or self-hypnosis) treatment to other types of therapy like stress management or psychotherapy show no convincing benefit for using hypnosis (Jacobson, 1973; Pekala, 2004).

Q: Can hypnosis cause sleep disorders?
A: There have been no documented hypnosis reports causing or leading to the development of a sleep disorder. There is a growing body of evidence that hypnosis can help with sleep disorders like insomnia (Borkovec, 1973), sleepwalking (Hurwitz, 1991), and sleep, terror.

Q: Is hypnotherapy a science?
A: Science is a method of acquiring knowledge; it's merely a process of putting your theories to the test to see whether they're backed up by evidence. Many researchers scientifically approach hypnosis study, generating research questions (hypotheses) and systematically evaluating them to see whether they are supported. Because of this, our understanding of hypnosis has advanced: previously, people believed that a mysterious magnetic fluid induced the effects of hypnosis; now, we believe that the effects are caused by a communication between the hypnotist and the subject, which can influence how the brain processes knowledge. Doctors and clinical psychologists are interested in hypnosis's impact on medical and psychological issues, while research psychologists are interested in what hypnosis is. Their research is published in journals, and you can use online resources like PubMed or Google Scholar to search the knowledge base. There are scientists interested in hypnosis, and you might assume that hypnosis is a science.

Hypnotherapy is the term we use to describe hypnosis to treat psychological and medical problems, and there is evidence that hypnosis can be used to treat illness. However, 'hypnotherapy is a controversial concept. Professional organizations such as the ESH, ISH, and ASCH believe that only qualified professionals (such as doctors, psychologists, dentists) should use hypnosis and use it as a tool alongside their other professional skills. Since hypnosis isn't considered therapy in its own right, a clinician would refer to themselves as "a doctor/dentist/psychologist who uses hypnosis" rather than "a hypnotherapist." People who call themselves hypnotherapists typically don't have any other healthcare credentials other than hypnotherapy training, and they don't publish much research. Given this, it's rational to believe that hypnotherapy is a science but that hypnotherapists don't contribute much to it.

Q: I frequently fall soundly asleep when using self-improvement hypnosis CDs. Are the CD's suggestions still reaching my subconscious mind, or is it blocked by the fact that I am sleeping and not in hypnosis?

A: During the 1950s, the idea of 'hypnopaedia,' or learning while sleeping, was popular. That is also when the majority of the study was completed. However, the findings do not appear to be very encouraging: one study by Emmons & Simon found that participants who'd been played recordings while sleeping did not perform any better than control participants in identifying words from a list. Since then, not much research has been done, suggesting that this is most likely not a fruitful research topic. More recent research has looked at whether or not people who are under general anesthesia will understand. In these experiments, very basic 'learning' is tested: far more basic than the kinds of deep level learning that a hypnosis CD could offer. The evidence indicates that very simple connections may be formed, but the complicated meanings of events are not fully understood (Deeprose, 2006). In conclusion, the evidence shows that hypnosis requires the participant to be awake.

Q: Under hypnosis, do people answer truthfully to the questions you ask?
A: They behave the same way they do when they are not hypnotized. People can't be compelled to do something they don't want to do, and they can't be forced to say the truth either. Because suggestions given during hypnosis may alter memories, whether purposely or accidentally, hypnotically-assisted memory retrieval is not admissible in court in most countries.

Q: Can negative behavior be induced under hypnosis without my free will?
A: See the previous response to the question of whether hypnosis would compel people to do things they don't want to do. The short answer is no: participants who are hypnotized have the right to refuse a suggestion in most situations.

Q: When do I start asking questions during a past life regression? I've seen REM and other trance symptoms several times, and I've asked questions, but they've either suddenly awakened or have already fallen asleep. When do I begin asking questions about childhood memories or past lives, and how do I do so?

A: I'm not sure what situation you're in, but unless you're adequately trained, I wouldn't ask questions about childhood memories or past lives while clients are hypnotized. While hypnosis is often used to revisit incidents from one's history, there is no evidence that it can help people remember childhood memories with any specific accuracy. When done incorrectly, you risk creating false memories, which can be particularly dangerous in patients who have undergone trauma. There is no scientific proof that past lives exist, and there is no evidence that incorporating the topic into therapy is effective. The only time I ever give past lives suggestions as a teaching method to explain how imaginative people's minds can be.

If clients/volunteers wake up or fall asleep unexpectedly and do not do so for the rest of the hypnosis session, I assume they are unhappy with what is going on and have not agreed to the process. I wouldn't recommend using regression methods unless you're sure you know what you're doing.

Q: I've learned that there are three types of people who are unhypnotizable: the drunk, the high on drugs, and can you tell me the third one?

A: The short answer is "people who do not want to be hypnotized," although there are a few myths to dispel. Hypnotisability is measured on a scale of one to ten; it does not mean that anyone can or cannot be hypnotized. "How hypnotizable is this person?" is a better question. Hypnotizability follows a normal distribution; a small percentage of people are 'highs,' a small percentage are 'lows,' and the rest will feel certain effects of suggestion in hypnosis. It is easy to become 'hypnotizable'; don't allow yourself to be hypnotized - no one can be hypnotized against their will. Surprisingly, certain substances, such as a nitrous oxide (laughing gas) and alcohol, tend to make people hypnotizable. However, it is based on the drug; others, such as diazepam, tend to have little effect.

Q: Is the idea of hypnosis being a special state of consciousness invalidated by highly motivated individuals faking hypnosis?
A: No more than claiming to have a broken leg invalidates the idea of a 'broken leg.' It's a fascinating phenomenon because it's possible to trick yourself into believing you're hypnotized. Stage hypnotists don't mind whether their subjects are faking or not as long as the audience is laughing. Researchers are having a tougher time distinguishing legitimate responses from fakers, but they have developed some innovative tools. Using the real/simulator design is one technique. The lows are told to act "as if" they are hypnotized in this design, and the highs are told to act "as if" they are hypnotized. If both groups perform equally, the outcome is unlikely to be due to hypnosis; however, if the highs perform differently, it's possible that some of the implied effects were true. The 'genuineness' of hypnotic effects has recently been examined using brain imaging techniques.

Q: Is hypnosis ever a one-session "quick fix" for a problem?

A: The answer to this question will be highly dependent on the nature of the 'problem.' It's easy to picture someone quitting smoking after a single session rather than healing from a more serious mental health condition like post-traumatic stress disorder (PTSD) or chronic depression.

In the case of smoking, some evidence shows that a proportion of people will abstain after only one hypnosis session. In one study, 23 percent of participants were still abstinent two years after a single hypnosis session. However, research shows that hypnosis is no more effective than other smoking cessation therapies, so a comparable proportion of people may be encouraged to stop smoking after only one session of either form of therapy, making hypnosis seem less special.

In the case of single-session therapies for other psychological issues, there does not seem to be any clear evidence for their effectiveness. There is a 'brief therapy' trend (often referred to as 'solution-focused brief therapy') that has proven beneficial for some conditions. Some therapists in the brief therapy movement are interested in 'single-session psychotherapy,' but there is very little monitored evidence that it is effective. In contrast to single-session therapies, there are hundreds of randomized controlled trials for cognitive-behavioral therapy for the treatment of psychological disorders. These controlled studies usually show that at least 6-20 sessions of psychotherapy are required to treat mild to moderate difficulties. CBT is commonly used in many financially constrained medical services worldwide to think more deeply about the context in which such therapy is administered. CBT is prescribed, which means that it is likely one of the most effective therapies available; treatment review bodies such as the Clinical Excellence and National Institute for Health agree with this evaluation. Brief therapy or single-session therapy is truly successful, practitioners must demonstrate it through controlled studies, which is yet to be demonstrated.

Q: Make individual differences in "imaginative suggestibility" provide a simpler explanation than dissociation in explaining responsiveness to hypnotic suggestions?

A: Dissociation theories of hypnosis propose that hypnosis causes 'splits' or dissociations of cognitive control systems. According to research, hypnotisability is higher in patients with 'dissociative' symptoms such as post-traumatic stress disorder. On the other hand, dissociation theories predict that stable people who dissociate more in everyday life would be more hypnotizable. This does not seem to be the case: research linking hypnotic suggestibility to dissociative experience scale (DES) scores have found no substantial correlation. Given this, it doesn't appear that dissociation is particularly useful in explaining hypnotic suggestion responsiveness.

Scores of inventive suggestibility (non-hypnotic suggestibility), on the other hand, have a strong correlation with hypnotic suggestibility (Kirsch & Braffman, 2001). This indicates a connection between the two, but there are two issues to address:

(1) Some people contend that the term "hypnosis" refers to a broad range of suggestions and that hypnotic and non-hypnotic suggestions are the same.

(2) Well, you may have explained why people react differently to hypnotic suggestions, but you haven't explained why people respond differently to non-hypnotic suggestions.

A theory to understand how people respond to non-hypnotic suggestions appears to be needed. Kirsch & Braffman (2001) argue that these factors include: attitudes towards hypnosis, response expectancy, absorption, fantasy proneness, and go/no-go reaction time. However, they caution that these variables don't account for all of the variability in non-hypnotic suggestibility. It's conceivable that there's an underlying ability to suggestibility, maybe with a genetic basis (Raz, 2008), or that there's a connection between suggestibility and the size of certain brain regions (Horton et al., 2004).

Q: Does the fact that highly motivated individuals can fake hypnotic effects invalidate the notion of hypnosis as a unique state of consciousness? Why, or why not?

A: Does the fact that a determined person can imitate a broken leg invalidate the concept of broken legs? Or does the fact that someone can fake depression invalidate the concept of depression? Because something can be faked does not make it any less real.

The "unique state of consciousness" is the part that I disagree with. It's difficult to distinguish between differentstates of consciousness from a scientific perspective. We're pretty good at determining whether someone is awake, asleep, or in a coma; however, science isn't so good at distinguishing between more subtle states of consciousness.

Rather than general 'states of consciousness,' more complex brain activity correlated with hypnosis and hypnotic effects can be considered. There is a lot of neuroimaging evidence to suggest that the effects of suggestion provided in hypnosis are unique and that they generate genuine effects. For example, a hypnotized individual given pain-relieving suggestions can experience less pain, which is linked to decreased activity in the network of brain regions involved in pain.

CONCLUSION

Weight and fitness are not always as good as we'd like to believe. When eating an unhealthy diet, you may be small. When practicing yoga, you can be overweight and go to the gym five days a week. Your physical appearance is not inherently linked to the way you are healthy. Losing weight doesn't mean you're getting full. Personal trainers also said: You can be overweight and healthy…

Being clinically obese will put you at a higher risk for type 2 diabetes, high cholesterol, high blood pressure, and even some cancer forms. However, making safe, sustainable decisions can have a huge effect on how you use your body through exercise and what you eat.

So, weight-loss hypnotherapy may be an option for others-gastric band hypnosis may offer a healthier alternative to surgery. In contrast, hypnotherapy can also help control emotional eating and recognize what may affect the food and weight relationship. This will help maybe that you have to go deeper than aesthetics.

It's time to focus on putting your mental health and wellbeing first, instead of focusing on how you look outside. It's time to dissect the quick solutions, solve the root issues, and make positive changes – not because of the time of year, pressure from friends or family, or what the media wants us to talk about.

CPSIA information can be obtained
at www.ICGtesting.com
Printed in the USA
LVHW080753160621
690358LV00007B/455

9 781802 102659